Intuitive Eating:

A revolutionary non-diet program to stop overeating, end your battle with food and find freedom from dieting forever. A workbook that works with tips to increase your health.

Table of Contents

Introduction: What Is Intuitive Eating?

Once you decide to be a little more health conscious, you are faced with a question constantly. That is "What should I eat?" Instead of stressing yourself out and pushing yourself an inch closer to eating the stress out, you can try a different kind of approach. That's what intuitive eating is for.

This is an excellent tool that encourages you to eat healthy. It can even help you end binging. It is not restricting.

You see, we all have an intuitive voice within us. And this voice can guide us to the right choices and the right portion sizes in food. What happens when we are bombarded with information about bad foods, good foods, bad portions, good portions, etc? We tamp down this intuitive voice. But it does not mean we cannot get it back. We can reconnect with this voice. We can reactivate our internal sense of fullness and hunger.

In a nutshell, intuitive eating is a different approach to dieting per se. It aims to help us foster a healthy relationship with our minds, bodies and food. It ultimately helps us become the master of our own bodies.

Intuitive eating teaches us to realize the difference between our emotional and physical feelings. We don't have to constantly worry about food, if you're eating a fattening food or not. The constant food worry ends here.

By getting a sense of our bodies, we learn to respond properly to the cues our inner bodies are sending us. The thing is we are all born with a natural intuition. We all know how to eat intuitively.

The challenge is uncovering the intuition because it is more likely tamped down by years and years, pile after pile of information from the media and the culture we are born into including dozens of influences, of food and diet myths.

There are no rigid healthy eating rules. Intuitive eating can be a challenge because it will ask you to dump what you have been fed all these years. To reactive your intuitive eating voice, you must forget all about what you know and have long known about food. You have to trust yourself. What awaits you is an unbelievable sense of freedom and satisfaction.

Chapter 1. Eating Disorders

What is an Eating Disorder?

The term eating disorder is used to describe an illness that is characterized by abnormal eating behavior and habits. These behaviors, in turn, cause severe changes and distress to the shape and weight of the body. A lot of people have misunderstood eating disorder to be an illness related to foods and lifestyle choices completely.

More than just disrupting your daily activities, this illness can affect your emotional and mental health. For instance, there could be times you find yourself feeling unduly anxious about your calorie intake or embarrassed about your weight. This may cause you to isolate from people, just for expressing their concerns about your health. The incident may generally lead to depression as a further symptom.

Generally, the more the illness is allowed to linger and not addressed, the more significant the damage caused, like affecting your digestion, the skin, bones, reducing teeth and gum strength, and even the heart performance.

There are different eating disorders out there that should not be taken lightly. They require attention and professional help. If you know someone who suffers from any of the known eating disorders, you should encourage them to seek medical care and give them emotional support that they need. Also, you need to be aware of the signs and symptoms of these disorders so that you know whether you are still on the health side or on the verge of suffering from them.

Binge Eating

This leads to eating enormous amounts of food even after the individual has had the feeling of a full stomach. Most people who suffer from binge eating try to hide it from friends and family, leading them to isolate themselves in many instances.

This is a similar eating disorder to Bulimia - with frequent loss of control overeating, but unlike Bulimia, there is no compensatory behavior afterward. From time to time everyone overeats, and so detecting this illness is somewhat complicated. However, when it becomes too often and frequent, not necessarily for hunger, it is a sign that it's not normal.

As a result, a lot of binge eating disorder patients end up obese. They are also at high risk of developing conditions that have to do with the cardio. Most of the times, binge eating disorder is usually accompanied or preceded by feelings of shame; also, intense feelings of emotions such as distress, embarrassment, and guilt. If not properly addressed, it further influences the progress of the condition. Binge eating by itself is not necessarily bad but becomes a disorder when the individual loses control overeating.

Other than emotions, there are kinds of foods you consume that help in triggering binge episodes. This is true of carbohydrates. Foods high in fats and carbohydrates, according to scientists can trigger the release of the serotonin hormone in the brain, which in turn induces pleasurable emotions and feelings. And binge eaters always tend to gravitate towards such.

Symptoms of this eating disorder include:

- A tendency to overeat because of loss of control

- Feelings of shame and guilt after overeating

- Binge eating without any compensatory behavior

- Consuming more food than intended

- Secretive about overeating

Food Addiction

Some people are addicted to food. They crave certain types of food and give in. They are not able to stop even when they are already full if they like the taste of the food. Overeaters and food addicts use food to achieve feelings of satisfaction. They often try to stop their food addiction, but just like other types of addicts, they often experience a relapse. Also, just like drug and alcohol addiction, food addiction can interfere with your life and put a strain on your relationships.

More often than not, people who binge eat or eat compulsively suffer from stress disorders and negative body image. Their stress can even stem from the disease itself. When you overeat, you may blame yourself for your actions, and this can make you stressed out afterward. When you are ashamed of your behavior, and you try to hide it from other people, you may become stressed out too. Again, your problems with overeating can make you more prone to overeating. It becomes a never-ending cycle.

Those who binge eat also tend to dislike the way they look. Their negative body image causes them to feel the need to eat less. Because they always worry about their physical appearance and the way other people think of them, they become stressed out. Also, their constant worry of eating more than they are supposed to make them stressed out even further. Such feelings of stress cause them to binge eat or feed their souls.

Then, there are others who just give up on themselves. They think that they are already fat, so why should they attempt to change their eating habits? They believe that it is hopeless for them to lose weight and be healthier. Some of them do not even exert effort only because, in their minds, their case is dropped already.

Emotional Eating

This is eating to fill emotional needs. Some people resort to eating whenever they feel stressed or sad. They think that if they eat the food they crave for during their time of stress, they will feel better. But most of the time, they feel even worse because they then become feel guilty for eating more than they should.

Eating emotionally is unhealthy. Besides it being a cause for being overweight, it doesn't let you address your right problem.

You may feel a little better while eating but when you finished your food, does it guarantee you that you will never feel stressed again? I mean, feeling stressed or sad or frustrated happens to anyone. I understand some people think it a little too often than others. You should deal with it the right way. You could use other diversions like watching movies or reading books, or you could ask for professional help on how to properly handle stress. If you continue this unhealthy habit, it could lead to obesity if you aren't already there. But it's never too late for you to change this pattern.

When you're emotionally hungry, you crave for specific comfort foods. Most of the time, these are unhealthy foods like junk foods or high-calorie foods like pizza and burger.

You don't get to pay attention and with what and how you eat. You don't thoroughly enjoy eating, you just eat and eat, and it takes time to feel full because it isn't your stomach that is hungry, it is your feelings.

Emotional hunger is sudden and often uncontrollable. You just feel it instantly, and you become powerless over it. Most people just give it to this craving right away.

Many of us do not make the connection between eating and our emotions. Understanding what drives us to indulge in emotional eating is a key factor to changing this unhealthy habit. A familiar myth we all have to disregard is about emotional eating being prompted by negative feelings like; stress, anxiety, anger or grief. Yes, people tend to eat bored, lonely, sad, stressed up or anxious. But, we all agree that at some point in life we have celebrated the good news with food. A child who grew up being given candy when they achieved something will continue doing so even when they grow up. This practice becomes their way of rewarding others too. Positive feeling contributes significantly to emotional eating; like on Valentine day, romantic desserts, popcorn and a bag of chips when watching a movie.

 About emotional eating, you have to remember that you are human, meaning that you're a passionate being. You have feelings, such as happiness, sadness, anger, and fear among others. This makes you prone to emotional eating, wherein you eat according to how you feel. More often than not, people eat to comfort themselves in times of despair or sorrow. You have to get rid of this habit and replace it with something healthier.

For example, whenever you are feeling down, you should go out for a jog. Being outdoors lets you breathe in fresh air. Jogging is an excellent way to raise your heart rate and exercise your body. Both of these are good for you because they relax you and make you feel good. More importantly, they keep you away from your refrigerator and prevent you from reaching for a tub of ice cream. When you eat comfort foods, you feel good at first.

Eventually, however, you start to regret your actions because you know that your body and health will pay for it in the end.

Furthermore, you have to get rid of your toxic and unhelpful nutritional beliefs. Do not be like those people who think that food is an enemy. Food is not your enemy. If you become fat, it is not the food's fault. It is your fault. If you harbor these beliefs, you will have an unhealthy relationship with food. So, you must change the way you think about food.

Identify Your Triggers

Although it is commonly known that emotional overeating is triggered by emotions; there are more specific factors that serve as triggers. Recognizing your personal triggers can greatly help you overcome emotional Causes and Symptoms of Emotional Eating

Emotional Eating is the process in which someone consumes a large amount of food, usually food that is unhealthy such as "junk foods," so that they could somehow feel better. In short, people afflicted with Emotional Eating Disorder use food as a means to alleviate the pain or loneliness that they are feeling.

Deal with Your Emotions

If your negative emotions are not dealt with in some way, you will continue on in an emotional eating frenzy. Even your positive emotions must have a creative outlet. Find other ways to celebrate a milestone or event besides eating. Going bowling or to see a movie is a celebration as well. Stay away from the popcorn unless you have saved room for it.

Denying that your emotions are an issue is not healthy, and, neither is ignoring your emotions. Ignoring a problem does not make it non-existent. It is fine to acknowledge those emotions. You can say, "I feel angry right now." You can say, "I am depressed today." Be honest about your emotions, but do not let them dictate you by going on a binge or lashing out at someone.

If your emotions are extremely out of control, seeing a counselor might be helpful. Not everyone who has emotional issues needs a counselor or therapy, but there is certainly nothing wrong with going for that type of help if it is needed. Whatever is needed to get you healthier is exactly what should be done if possible.

In some societies, people have not been taught to deal with what is difficult or challenging. While this might seem pleasant, it is hardly helpful. Many children and adults have not been taught to allow themselves to feel and work through the unpleasant emotions.

If you are angry, acknowledge the anger. Feel it, but do not let it spin out of control. If you are sad, go through the experience, but do not stay there. If you are depressed, allow yourself to feel the emotion, then, deal with it. Is there a legitimate reason to feel depressed such as a loss or major change in life? If not, then it could be an issue that requires medical help. Mindfulness does not encourage denying the emotion. You are encouraged to face it and deal with it.

If you are stressed out, look at the cause of the stress. If something can be eliminated from your life, then remove it. If it is a situation that you are unable to walk away from, then you must have a strategy to deal with the situation. Counselors are a good source for those types of strategies. In the meantime, you can still practice mindful eating so that the issue does not spill over into your eating habits any more than it already has.

Overeating and Under-Eating

Both over and under-eating is a significant problem for many individuals. Society leads us to believe that being skinny is the only acceptable "norm" which causes many people to diet excessively and this mainly affects young girls and women.

This leads to what we call under-eating, as people then tend to cut down on certain foods or even a variety of foods, with the primary goal being to lose weight or to maintain the low body weight which they are happy with.

However, we need to remember that we cannot all look the same (or be that skinny) as each person is different, our body shapes are different, and our body's needs are very different. Thus, you need to do what is best for you and your optimum level of health.

The same applies to overeating, as we seem to spend more and more time at work and less time cooking healthy meals. The result of this is that the fast food industry is making more money than ever before. A lot of people tend to grab fast foods, as this is the more convenient and more accessible route to follow.

This is also where overeating comes into play, as people may work out on the road or miss a meal here and there, which results in overeating when they do get to enjoy a meal. It is exceptionally effortless to overeat when one eats too fast.

Although we are not mentioning that we should not eat any fast food at all, the fact remains that fast foods are not necessarily the healthiest meal and unfortunately too much fast food can lead to weight and health issues also.

We need to continue cooking and eating healthy mindful meals and cut the fast-food habit down to a mindful eating "treat" which one may look forward to. Eating everything in moderation is the key to happy and healthy life. Overeating is a common problem. However, it is a straightforward concept. Some people think that they overheat due to a weak willpower. They believe that they cannot control their appetite, and it is why they cannot lose any weight. The truth is that they do not have a problem with their willpower. They are merely overeaters who do not eat when they eat. What does this mean?

When you do not eat when you eat, you are not wholly present during your meal. You are not fully aware of how it tastes or how it nourishes your body. Your brain misses out on a vital phase of nutritional experience, which involves satisfaction and taste. Your mind either thinks that it did not eat enough or it did not eat at all. So, you think that you are hungry and you eat more than you are supposed to. If you want to avoid overeating, see to it that you increase your presence and awareness during mealtime.

Also, there is this misconception that when you eat quickly, you boost your metabolism. The truth is that eating slowly helps you boost your metabolism. When you eat fast, you put stress on your body. Keep in mind that humans are just not biologically designed for high-speed eating. If you eat quickly, you put your body into a physiologic stress response. This, in turn, causes decreased nutrient assimilation, digestion, and calorie burning rate. Conversely, it causes increased appetite and nutrient excretion.

When you slow down, you improve your nutritional metabolism. You also get to taste your food better, which heightens your satisfaction. You need to increase your pleasure in eating to enjoy it more. You do not have to eat more of the food. You just have to take some time to appreciate its taste, presentation, and overall quality. Pleasure catalyzes a relaxation response as well as fuels assimilation and digestion. What's more, you get the chance to chew your food more carefully. You can make sure that you can digest it properly.

Anorexia Nervosa

Anorexia nervosa is a psychological wellbeing disease as. Individuals with this issue have a serious distraction with sustenance and self-perception. They don't eat, count calories too much, or generally eat awfully little to look after wellbeing. Regardless of being underweight, they frequently have tension concerning the conviction that they are overweight and keep on trying to shed pounds. While the condition is more typical in young ladies, it is currently accepted to influence more young men and Women than beforehand thought. Measurements demonstrate that anorexia frequently begins between 13-30 years old.

Its symptoms include excessive weight loss, avoidance of eating enough to retain a healthy weight, a wrong perception of one's looks and anxiety towards gaining weight and becoming obese. Often the patient begins subjecting him/herself to excessive diets, resulting in rapid loss of weight. But often patients continue refusing to eat even when their weight is below normal. Because of a distorted perception of their looks, anorexics think they still aren't as thin as they should be and continue dieting. Their anxiety not to become obese drives them to excessive exercise, the use of purgatives and minimal consumption of food. Slowly, this pattern acquires the characteristics of fixation and often approaches the point of the possibility of starving.

Even though these are not always related to the disorder, we present some of the signs that appear in cases of anorexia:

Mental Signs

• Mental fixation overeating and one's weight

• A distorted perception of one's looks

• Self-esteem defined by one's weight and appearance

• Highly self-judgmental attitude and perfectionism

Psychological signs

• Clinical depression

• Low idea of one's self

• Mood swings

Social Signs

• Avoiding contact with friends

• Worsening of relationship with family

• Productivity and engaging with work or assessments facing severe decline (however, because of perfectionism this isn't always the case)

Signs in Behavior

• Excessive exercise or training

• Refusal to eat and obsession with calories intake

• Secretive behavior concerning food and weight

• Self-harm, tendencies towards suicide, excessive use of drugs

In men, anorexia often manifests together with psychological issues and often follows a time period during which they have been obese. Male anorexics also often have a distorted perception of the way they look.

In women, the signs of anorexia appear in relation to a general state of unhappiness regarding their own body and an obsession with becoming as thin as possible. Female anorexics often demonstrate patterns of excessive perfectionism.

Aside from the mental symptoms, anorexia's bodily signs in those of young age are related to their growth and development. A person's daily life is greatly affected; their interest in activities they used to enjoy obviously deteriorates. A number of sufferers also demonstrate the signs of clinical depression.

Even though anorexia is defined as "lack of appetite," anorexics often don't lose their appetite. They enjoy eating and do feel hunger, but they don't think about eating like everybody else, which can be observed in a great number of different behaviors. To provide examples, they are prone to lying regarding their food consumption, providing excuses for refusing to eat, claiming they have already eaten when they haven't, and concealing how much weight they have really lost, and so on.

If malnourishment or the possibility of starvation has begun to affect your body, medical measures will have to be taken. Doctors treat conditions that are the result of anorexia nervosa such as osteoporosis, a heart condition, or clinical depression. As you begin to recover, a doctor will carry on monitoring your health and maintain you at a healthy weight.

Bulimia Nervosa

Bulimia is an eating disorder identified by consistent bouts of overeating which are directly followed by vomiting, the use of diuretics and purgatives or enemas. In the majority of cases, bulimia sufferers hide their actions because they feel guilty of gluttony. Bulimics understand that their eating behavior isn't normal. Bulimia nervosa constitutes a very risky condition since the signs of the problem aren't obvious and a diagnosis is very difficult to make.

Bulimics don't necessarily have weight issues. They sometimes have normal weight. The obsessive wish to lose weight, triggered by mental or emotional issues, doesn't allow them control of their bulimic episodes. If they throw up the same amount of food as they have consumed, their bodies suffer from malnourishment which can result in significant loss of weight, yet this isn't always the case.

Bulimia nervosa manifests itself most among women between the ages of fifteen and thirty. The last stage of bulimia nervosa is the demonstration of major clinical depression, which can result in the sufferer committing suicide.

One may make many attempts to lose weight by subjecting oneself to severe diets. The bulimic's weight ranges around normal and can be five kilos more or less between times of excessive eating and times of dieting. Individuals suffering from bulimia nervosa are often anxiously worried, depressed or demonstrate mood swings. Bulimia in a great number of cases works together with anorexia and it is often difficult to identify which of them is the more prevalent.

Here are several signs that can assist you in identifying someone who might have developed bulimia nervosa:

- Bad teeth, from stomach acids during vomiting;

- Visiting the toilet after eating (to secretly throw up);

- Wounded fingers, due to being pushed into the throat for vomiting;

- Weakness, exhaustion or fainting;

- Dehydration;

- Malfunctions of the heart;

- Sore mouth and throat;

- Disruption or disorders in the menstrual period;

- Frequently eating too much, particularly fattening foods; Dealing with bulimia nervosa

- First, understand the existence of the problem.

- Discuss the issue with someone, without expecting them to judge you.

- Stay away from individuals who can only talk about food and diets.

- Understand that you can assume control over your eating habits.

- Ask for the help of professional or discuss it with a psychologist.

- Get advice concerning the disorder.

- Remember that your weight is healthy, particularly when you feel the need to get rid of food you have consumed.

- Create a plan to cope with emotional problems and depression.

- Seek positive role models whom you can relate to, to assist you in increasing your self-esteem. Remember that projected mass media thin models or actors often represent unhealthy lifestyles.

- Acquire regular eating habits and do not subject yourself to diets.

Chapter 2. Benefits of Intuitive Eating

It is obvious you look good when you are healthy, which is the state intuitive eating helps you achieve, but that is not all that you enjoy. Once you get into the habit of intuitive eating, making it your lifestyle, there are many more benefits that accrue to you. However, before we get there, it is important to ensure you know how to distinguish real hunger from cravings.

How to Distinguish Real Hunger from Cravings

Probably you are into the habit of reaching out for snacks when you are idle or bored, and it is possible you eat a lot when you are annoyed with someone or upset about something. Those, right there, are wrong reasons for eating, and because you are so used to using food in that manner, you might find it difficult to tell when the urge to eat is out of a physical need by your body, or other extraneous reasons.

•   If you are ashamed of yourself every time you eat, then, chances are you are reaching out to food when you are not genuinely hungry.

•   If you find yourself eating too quickly and not finding the need to chew, chances are that your physical body is not the one demanding to be fed.

•   If you have felt like eating only after a stressful situation, chances are there is an emotional need seeking to be attended to but disguising itself as hunger.

- If you have been feeling like eating too often even after you have had major meals, chances are that what you are consuming is not for the benefit of your physical body.

- If after a meal you experience the stuffed feeling, it is likely you have exceeded the amount your physical body requires, or you probably ate when you were actually not hungry in the real sense of the word.

- If you think you are hungry and the first instinct is to go for some vegetables, nuts or fruits, you are very likely, experiencing genuine hunger. On the contrary, if you think you are hungry and the first thing that comes to mind is ice-cream, chocolate, doughnuts or confectionaries, you are very likely just bored or in need for consolation of sorts. The latter foods mostly satisfy cravings and no matter how much of them you eat, the sense of hunger is not likely to disappear.

Once you have learnt to understand the language of your body and get used to responding to it appropriately, eating intuitively will become a part of your everyday life. In the process you will enjoy:

(1)♟♟♟ Enhanced digestion

The key points you need to remember as far as intuitive eating is concerned are:

> (i)♟♟ *The importance of eating when you are genuinely hungry*

(ii) ♟♟♟♟♟♟♟♟♟♟♟ *The importance of eating until the hunger is gone – till you are satisfied. This part excludes eating until you feel stuffed.*

As long as you are observing those two fundamental points, your digestive system will not be overloaded with amounts of sugar, fat and salt it finds difficult to process and dispose of.

One of the biggest victims when you overstuff your body with food or keep eating without a break is the liver, because it has to keep working at filtering toxins from those foods and to digest the fat. Of course your stomach will also be on an overdrive, because every time you eat something, it has to pump out more enzymes as well as acids to work on it. In short, once you are practicing intuitive eating, your body has some time to rest before the next genuine hunger strikes.

Intuitive eating keeps you from problems of digestion that emanate from loading freshly consumed food onto partially digested food. When you subject your digestive system to such a scenario, it gets confused as what digestive stage it should be subjected the food to. No wonder people who eat haphazardly and without regard to genuine hunger keep complaining about constipation, indigestion and such other digestion related problems.

(2)♟♟ Reduced incidences of stress

It has been noted that intuitive eaters do not suffer as much emotional stress as people making a conscious effort to diet and lose weight. Owing to the freedom intuitive eaters enjoy and the luck of pressure regarding what, how much and when to eat, they are usually in a good mood free of stress. They are usually emotionally healthier than their counterpart dieters who are generally plagued with anxiety and depression. In fact, a good number of people from the latter group engage perennially in negative self-talk, and that only jeopardizes their chance of success in their dieting program.

On the contrary, when these same dieters switch to intuitive eating, they are less tense and anxious, and soon their psychological welfare significantly improves. There are various reasons why dieters experience stress as opposed to people who eat intuitively, but one of the main ones is the fact that they allow themselves to relax and enjoy the meal, rather than concentrating on analyzing the make-up of the food and its weight in terms of calories. Every time you are warning yourself to stop reaching out for this food item solely to fight body weight, it is a sure way of building stress. Minus such caveats, you are so relieved that your body no longer craves what you have sworn not to give it; because there is nothing like that, anyway.

(3)♟♟ Reduction and stabilization of weight

For you as an intuitive eater, you have no fear of failing, because you do not have a set target for your weight. So, you have nothing to be disappointed about any day. Instead, you have left your body to dictate what it needs, and you feed it accordingly. In any case, when you dictate a set amount of food for morning or lunch, for instance, and the challenges of the body probably vary from day to day, is it not probable that you will end up overstuffing your body sometimes while starving it at other times?

Because in intuitive eating you heed your body's language and feed it only what it requires, your body ends up settling at an optimal weight. It has actually been noted that people practicing intuitive eating often have favorable BMIs.

There is also the aspect of intuitive eating being responsible for a stress-free environment while direct dieting contributes to a rise in stress level. Biologically, it has been observed that the hormone, cortisol, which is associated with stress, is also responsible for weight gain. In short, people who get on regulated weight-loss programs end up involuntarily jeopardizing their chances of success by the stressful environment they find themselves in.

(4)⚜ Strengthening self esteem

There are few things as bad as setting a goal, as you do in dieting, and failing miserably. Of course, simply having that in mind can be a source of anxiety, and every time you think about failing you contemplate eating less. Suppose you are eating less when your body genuinely needed more, what message do you think you will be passing to it? The body will understand you to mean there is scarcity of food, and therefore it had better not utilize everything you gave it before.

Can you see how that can sabotage your efforts at losing weight? Your body slows down its metabolism and hoards some calories it would, otherwise have burnt, and when you gain weight despite your efforts to eat less, you get frustrated and probably deem yourself a failure. Hence your self-esteem drops and you are in a bad place emotionally. What do people suffering emotionally do? They reach out for comfort foods, among other unhealthy habits. What about when you eat at will like in intuitive eating and yet you keep losing unhealthy weight? Your self-esteem rises, you become a happier you, and you even gain more friends. Happy people with a positive outlook to life attract similar friends. In the social arena, this is how the law of attraction works.

(5)♟♟ Enhanced body awareness

Once you become used to intuitive eating, listening to your body becomes automatic. You will even read your body when it is low in, say, iron, and be in a position to remedy the situation without the need to see a physician for more technical and expensive interventions.

In short, in intuitive eating, you do not only read your body's signs of hunger and satiety, you also read its signs in totality. For that reason, you are able to address each sign in the most relevant way, as opposed to cases where people turn to food to suppress the signs extraneous to hunger. Intuitive eaters are not going to serve a bowl of food just because they feel exhausted even after resting all day. They will very likely appreciate that the composition of meals they have eaten for sometime has been short on vegetables and other sources of iron, and to remedy that they are going respond with lots of vegetable salads. Most likely, the body itself is going to yearn for those foods and will not let you leave the butchery or meat store without a piece of liver.

This is an advantage conventional dieters do not enjoy, as they are not intent on listening to their bodies. That is the reason weight loss is not necessarily tantamount to good health. You can consume the same amount of calories with an intuitive eater and be lethargic while the intuitive eater remains energetic because of heeding the body's call of relevant foods. With the intuitive eater, the name calorie does not feature anywhere. It is all about – how do I feel?

Chapter 3. Emotional Hunger Versus Physical Hunger

Right from infancy, we have been taught to identify hunger as the need for nourishment. The need for food. After all, food keeps us alive. The nutrients from food replace our worn out tissues. We know the basics of how the digestive system works. We learned we are to eat three square meals in a day to sustain ourselves. But that isn't even anywhere near the truth. Our ancestors never ate three meals a day. We weren't designed that way.

Now it's even worse, because we have so much junk food available on demand. There's at least two or three fast food joints around the corner. We're a society that's gone food crazy! We're always supersizing this or that. It's nuts!

So allow me at this point to address the difference between TRUE physical hunger, and emotional hunger. Because it's only when you understand the difference that you'll be able to better handle yourself the next time you think of hitting that Taco Bell again.

Physical Hunger

True physical hunger is when your body pressingly demands food. It's undeniable. You stomach feels like an empty black hole. You might get a touch dizzy or light-headed. Sometimes you get nauseous. You can't really focus on the task at hand. You get so easily irritated, like, "Why does the air smell like air? What the hell?"

At that moment you know you have to eat something, and the sooner you do it, the better too. In other words, physical hunger is something you actually feel. There are actually physical effects. None of it is in your head.

All this is made possible by a hormone called ghrelin. Ghrelin is secreted by the stomach, brain, pancreas, and the small intestine. While it's responsible for many things in the human body, for now, we are only interested in its function as the "hunger hormone."

You see, ghrelin is what tells the brain you know you need to open your piehole and shove some damn pies in. It increases a person's appetite and food absorption and is responsible for fat storage in humans.

When we are short of energy in the body, ghrelin is produced in the stomach walls, and then transmits a signal to the brain to increase appetite and food intake. It also plays a huge role in body mass.

Ghrelin has an arch nemesis called leptin. Who knew there was so much drama going on in your body, right? Anyway, leptin does the opposite of what ghrelin does. What's that? You guessed it. It reduces the appetite. Thin people are said to have lower amounts of ghrelin and higher leptin levels, while the reverse is the case for overweight people.

Those are the basics of physical hunger. So, next time your stomach growls, take it seriously because it's an emergency!

Emotional Hunger

Emotional hunger is all in your mind. Sometimes you might feel like you have a yawning ache inside you that nothing else can satisfy. Some might say what you are experiencing is emotional hunger. It is a very common thing to experience. Either way, emotional hunger can be really hard to beat, especially when you've indulged in it so much you now emotionally eat on autopilot. But you can beat it! You *know, mind over matter!*

On Emotions

It's natural to feel emotions. That's a huge part of our shtick as humans. Emotions matter, and are important. You need to pay as much attention to them as you would the food you eat, or the job you do.

That is why we have to be cognisant of our habits and what issues cause us to be dependent on comfort foods. Once you are able to deal with the issues, give yourself a reality check. As a human, you have intelligence beyond compare. That level of intelligence gives you the ability to be a problem solver. But what good is intelligence without emotions? Even Siri has emotions! The emotions stop us from being totally robotic with needed attributes like empathy, compassion, love and the like.

34

Whatever it is you might have suffered emotionally; you can focus positive energy into getting better. It may just last longer than you want. But you will surely get better.

Emotional Hunger Triggers

Emotional hunger is easy to identify if you know what you are looking for. Have you been told by a friend or lover that you are too clingy? That you call too much? You have tried not to, but you can't seem to help yourself. Those are signs you are looking for emotional assurance. Signs you are afraid to be left alone.

When you act like this, you are more likely to read meanings where there are none. You feel hurt when people do not act the way you expect them to act or the way you envisioned them reacting. Once things don't go the way you planned, you go on an emotional decline which causes you to eat emotionally to satisfy your emotional hunger.

Because it feels like food is the only thing that doesn't judge you.

But it doesn't have to be so!

Overthinking

Emotionally hungry people are of the opinion they know what's in everybody's head, that they know what everybody is thinking and saying about them. Vying for acceptance among people and attention based solely out of the conclusions you have jumped to is a recipe for disaster. Why? When you get disappointed, your emotional belly is triggered, and next thing you know, you're three-quarters through a 1 litre tub of Ben and Jerry's.

One major characteristic of emotionally hungry people is trying to conform to certain ideologies or behaviors that have been deemed acceptable by a group of people so as not to be left out or hanging.

Self-Loathing and Dissatisfaction

More often than not, emotionally hungry people try to look, behave, talk or dress like other people. Mostly people with high profile social status. These people they want to have what the emotionally hungry person has tried unsuccessfully to get. A lot of friends, adoring fans, a great figure, six packs and muscles, a good job, an awesome ability to stick to diets, etc.

Most emotionally hungry people are often heard saying, "How I wish I could be like this person; she doesn't have to watch what she eats"

"How I wish I could look like that; I could wear whatever I wanted!" The more they wish, the sadder they become, and the weaker their resolve gets and the more they eat emotionally.

The whole concept of emotional hunger is the need to feel something different from the same old boring stuff. The need to "feel alive."

Ways People Deal with Emotional Hunger

While some eat emotionally to deal with these feelings, many others engage in more activities like sports to feel alive, and this in turn satisfies their emotional hunger. This is a great thing!

For others who crave human contact, they have sex - not necessarily to bond with the other person, but to feel whatever it is they want to feel. For most people, casual sex is completely acceptable. An emotionally hungry person will see it as more than just fun, though. To them, casual sex is a form of "nourishment." They avoid serious emotions that make them seem emotionally inadequate, choosing to go thrill seeking. This is them just trying to feel like they are good enough.

It's not their fault! In a purely judgmental society where a person can't be fit enough, slim enough, beautiful enough, or plainly good enough, they feel like they don't fit anywhere. Sex feels like the easiest way to make ourselves believe we have gotten our emotional hunger satisfied.

It's Not Enough Though

After some time, that too doesn't work or it feels like it doesn't work as well as it used to. At that moment we feel like we are getting approval from that one person we are interacting with. We feel we are good enough. We feel no other person's opinion matters. We feel we are worthy of another person's attention mixed with the "feel good" hormones secreted by the brain after sex. We seem satisfied at that moment and every other person's opinion seems inconsequential because we feel "good."

If you can relate, then you know chances are you are prone to having more sex partners than is healthy. Let's not even forget the fact there are enough STDs going around to get you in some hot water sooner or later.

Sex and Emotional Pain

Although research has found sex eases the pain, sadness, and anger one feels against something; it's not exactly a long lasting solution to the underlying problem. While you can and should explore your sexuality in healthy ways, you should not be doing so as a way to cope with unhealthy emotions. Sadly, this is what the majority of people do. Research shows a majority of people who engage in random and casual sex are trying to feed an emotional hunger. Trying to prove they are good enough.

If you feel you can't go through recovering from emotional hunger on your own, you could always look for a trusted relative, or a friend. If you find despite the support systems you have available, beating this is a struggle, then don't be afraid or ashamed to seek out professional help.

Drugs and Emotional Hunger

Similar to sex, people turn to drug use as a coping mechanism for emotional hunger. This is very common in people who are trying to numb their pain. It may be the pain of loss, the pain of a broken home or even physical pain.

There a lot of short-term fixes people use when they do not know how to satisfy their emotional hunger. Some are very self-destructive methods, like drug abuse and alcohol. Others feel socially awkward so they would rather remain in isolation and adapt to their own company instead of interacting with others and risk being treated wrongly.

When you feel like you have lost all control of yourself. When you lose your ability to moderate your use of certain substances, or when you notice you are using these substances only to satisfy your emotional needs, it would be advisable to seek help from a therapist or doctor.

To most emotionally hungry people, the idea of being single or out of a relationship can be really scary. To avoid or lose that feeling of loneliness, you will most likely do things that are not good for your health. Things you feel will be able to fill that gaping emotional hole you are so scared of.

Emotional Hunger Triggered by Breakups
Most emotionally hungry people in relationships react very badly to an idea of a break up. They never feel like there is a problem and most times refuse to believe they are the cause of the problem. These people have a very difficult time accepting rejection.

Since emotionally hungry people often seek acceptance and proximity with people, they usually do not know how to respect boundaries, because they find it difficult.

Dealing with emotional hunger is wholly about working with your mind, and reprogramming yourself to deal with issues in a healthier manner. Keep friends who are ready to invest as much energy into your relationship as you do.

So, we have ascertained that emotional hunger doesn't necessarily have to do with emotional eating all the time, but it can quickly progress into that if other methods of solace do not work for you.

Now, let's tackle this head on.

Chapter 4. Distracting Yourself

Distracting Alternatives to Eating

Recognizing that your urge to eat in a way which is contrary to your diet plan is your primitive brain giving voice to its survival drives, and then choosing to ignore it will necessarily mean that you refrain from emotional eating.

But if that's all you do you risk being in an endless loop where you have the urge to eat, realize that it is your primitive brain and not you which wishes to eat, and ignore it repeated over and over again.

You don't eat, which is good, but it's not a pleasant way to pass the time and if that's all you do there is a risk that you will eventually grow weary of it and eat something just to shut it up.

To avoid that unfortunate scenario you can choose, once you recognized the voice of your primitive brain, and made the decision to ignore it, to distract yourself with some other activity than eating and thus obtain some peace.

We all know what it feels like to be so involved with something that we forget to eat. We miss a meal or two or more without even realizing that we are hungry.

Distracting ourselves, when we have the urge to engage in emotional eating works on much the same principle. We forget about eating because we're distracted by something sufficiently engaging to retain our attention.

The key to distracting activities is that they be relatively passive and easy to implement. They must be readily available, take no particular effort or expenditure of energy, and the activities which you enjoy or at least find reasonably palatable.

They should also be activities to which a default out of habit, rather than new activities which you do rarely, or which you do because you think you should.

In other words, it's okay for you to distract yourself by reading fiction if that's something you habitually do as a distraction or escape. But you shouldn't attempt to distract yourself with War and Peace, or Moby Dick, if you don't ordinarily read literature.

An important caveat: be wary of engaging in a distracting activity which you tend to do while eating. For example, if you tend to numb out watching television with a plate of cookies, watching television may not be an ideal distraction for you.

If you can't find any distraction in the list below which you don't associate with eating, and can't come up with any similar activities of your own that don't involve food, then you should look for soothing alternatives instead.

It's likely, however, you will be able to find a distracting alternative which you don't associate with eating.

Remember, these distracting activities are fallbacks for when you don't have the energy to engage in better options.

You may never need to use them, but give yourself permission to if you can't muster up the strength or motivation to use the better options presented later.

There's a good chance that you won't need passive distractions from thoughts of food once you've learned to use EEESY™ to soothe and quiet your primitive brain, and as you progress with it you almost certainly won't.

But in the meantime give yourself permission to veg out if that's all you can manage.

Distracting activities

1. Watching television. This is the first on the list as, for many people, it meets all of the requirements noted above. It takes no effort, is readily available, and it's something we typically resort to take our minds off things.

It's completely passive, and can be quite enjoyable particularly with the wide range of viewing options currently available.

Although we often associate television watching with eating here's a trick that may help you resist food cravings while watching TV: watch something incompatible with eating, something that will put you off food, like a horror movie or documentary about disease. It's also good if you can watch something without commercials which often advertise food.

If this is a distracting activity which appeals to you, it's a good idea to ensure you have programming available which you like.

If you need a distraction while you are already watching TV — and this is bound to happen — choose one from the remainder of the list.

2. Reading. There is no such thing as a trashy novel, if it can transport you to a fictional world far from the cares and worries of the real one.

There are worse habits to have than reaching for a romance novel on a Friday night — when you are too tired from a busy work week to do anything requiring more effort — and escaping through fiction rather than food.

3. Playing video games. You may not have a regular Halo night, but if you enjoy playing video games there's nothing wrong with using them as a distraction.

4. Internet activities. This could include surfing the Internet, participating in virtual worlds such as Second Life, engaging in online forums, or other online activities.

Yes, you're wasting time, but as long as you're not eating when you're online it can be a compelling and thus beneficial distraction from food.

Chapter 5. How to Succeed at Intuitive Eating and Avoid Common Mistakes

re you ready to begin your journey to intuitive eating? The process is straight forward but takes some practice to adapt to your body and needs. Set goals for yourself: learn to read your body's signals and communication. Review your schedule to make sure you have enough time during the day to eat if you feel hungry, and set aside room for exercise, relaxation, and meditation. This section will focus on errors and common mistakes that can hinder your progress in maintaining a healthy success with mindful eating.

Avoid Skipping Meals

This is good advice for anyone. Skipping meals is sometimes inevitable, especially if your schedule doesn't allow much time to take a break. If you expect this to happen and can prepare ahead, get up early to start breakfast early. Pay attention to your level of hunger in the morning, to determine how much you want to eat. Bring a light snack to work or school, just in case there is an opportunity to satisfy your hunger, should you feel this way and need to prolong or skip lunch. Whether you eat small or large meals, ensure that you have something nutritious and tasty, just in case. Even the best-planned schedules can change at the last minute, and being prepared can alleviate a lot of unnecessary stress.

Not Drinking Enough Water

Hunger can be a symptom of dehydration. If you feel hungry, drink water first. Being hydrated is one of the most important ways to stay healthy. It can also regulate your hunger signals so that when you feel like eating, it is a response to hunger and not for other reasons. If drinking water during the day doesn't appeal to you, try adding lemon, lime or cucumber. Sparkling water can be another alternative. Herbal teas are great during colder months, to ensure you are hydrated. Fruit contains a lot of water and natural sugar, which can provide a boost in energy in between meals if needed. Coffee is acceptable in moderation, though alternate drinking coffee with water, as it can have a dehydrating effect.

Setting Unrealistic Goals

Many of us set goals when we diet, and often, they can be unrealistic. Magazines, advertisements and diet programs promote quick fixes and sure-fire ways to lose weight fast, but this is only good in the interim. In extreme cases, where weight loss is necessary for health reasons, a medical professional or nutritionist may provide a specific guideline for eating. Even within this plan, mindful eating can be practiced, by noticing how the food you eat impacts you and when you eat. Choosing healthy foods can be counter-productive if we eat when we're not hungry or too much when we are, therefore not listening to our signals.

Focus on one goal at a time, if necessary, to avoid discouragement and disappointment. In other words, don't expect to lose a lot of weight, reduce your anxiety and lower your sugar levels all at once, though if you eat relatively healthy and exercise, even moderately, you'll likely see positive results within a few weeks. The key is not to expect overnight transformations that you can post on social media for a shocking response. Even the most successful people, when it comes to losing one hundred pounds or becoming athletic, must dedicate months, even years, to achieving their goals. When the goal is reached, maintenance is still needed and must continue. Mindfulness can instill that level of maintenance from the very beginning so that it becomes part of your everyday way of living.

Obstacles to Intuitive Eating: Emotional Response to Food and Changing Habits

We all have habits that are difficult to break or change, and it's not something that can be achieved overnight. Recognizing a negative habit is a start to making an improvement, as it shows we are aware of it. Habit forming traits often happen as a response to something else in our life. For example, we may overeat when we feel emotionally upset or as a way to make ourselves feel better when we have a challenging experience. This can happen when someone is grieving or feeling a sense of loss. Food can often take the place of that loss in order to cope. When you are going through a difficult time, it's important to not blame yourself, especially for eating habits. Realize that it is temporary, and in time, when you are ready, you can change the way you think about eating. The key is awareness. A helpful approach is a meditation, to give yourself that space to reflect, without judgment, and set realistic goals.

Avoid Multi-Tasking When You Eat

Meeting a deadline, chatting online or in person, and getting work done are all activities that many people try to accomplish during a meal. This happens most often during lunch break, as a "working lunch" or as a way to save time and alleviate the stress of having to complete the work after lunch, though the opposite will occur. As you try managing both tasks, your eating habits and connecting with your body's signals will interfere. This breaks the connection between your food and you. It is during this multi-tasking that you may feel more anxious to rush back to work from lunch, or in a more social and conversational atmosphere, lose that sensation you experience when you enjoy your meal alone and without distraction. Even if you are pressed for time, leaving a minimum of twenty minutes to enjoy a meal is a good start. Put down the files, leave the computer screen and go for a walk in a quiet and serene place. Meals, whenever you choose to enjoy them and when you can find adequate time and space for them, should take center stage, and all other events put on pause until you are finished.

If you enjoy eating with co-workers, family, and friends, make it an enjoyable event. Keep it positive and fun. If a working lunch is what you want to do, find that enjoyment in your food when you can and chew, savor every mouthful. Keep multi-tasking to a minimum, if you have to keep tasks in motion during your break. Your team may notice how you slow down to eat and enjoy the taste of your food. It may be appropriate to talk about the food and appreciate what you have. This may encourage others to see how you approach intuitive eating and could motivate them as well!

What is Emotional Eating? How to Identify and Cope With Emotional Eating Habits

Emotional eating can best be defined as a response to eating as a means of coping with stress and difficult situations in life. This can become chronic, in order to fill in a void or gap in our life that we have challenges dealing with. In some cases, where this becomes a recurring and extreme, eating disorders may result. For most people, it's a sign that we are responding to stress, grief and other feelings with food, even when we do not experience hunger. This results in a pattern of binge-eating or over-eating and in some cases, going without food for a while, until hunger pangs become unbearable, causing us to overeat. In extreme cases, bulimia or anorexia are examples of eating disorders that cause us to avoid food (anorexia) or bounce between eating too much, then forcing yourself to eliminate food and lose weight (bulimia).

Food can represent more than nourishment. It is seen as a reward, a coping mechanism or comfort. The term "comfort food" signifies the needs for food as a way to deal with a hardship, such as a relationship break up, losing a job or a sense of failure when an expectation isn't met. It's counterproductive in the long-term, but it makes us feel good right away. Movies and television shows will sometimes show a character binging on a tub of ice cream after breaking up with their partner. This is an emotional response to a difficult experience.

Growing up, we learn to associate food with different aspects of our life. A lollipop or ice cream cone as a reward for good behavior or an extra slice of cake for helping with chores. It can also be restrictive, even punitive when portions or types of food are limited if we were pressured to lose weight and eat a certain way. There may be positive intentions to both, but ultimately, we learn from childhood to see food as a tool to reward, punish or comfort. It's not an easy pattern to reverse, though it can be done by acknowledging these traits have been ingrained into us at a young age and recognizing the response to food when we experience one of these in adulthood:

A reward as an adult may entail having an extra slice of cake to reward good eating habits during the first week of a diet
A punishment may be restricting what you eat over the next month, to make up or "correct" a binge or period of time where you ate foods considered forbidden by following a diet
Choosing to eat to cope with the grief of loss, stress or frustration from occurrences in life

What is the first sign of emotional eating? Cravings! These are common and we experience them daily. Cravings occur even when you are not hungry, as a response to an event. For example, if you feel stressed at work, you may crave chocolate or a bag of chips. The flavor may be appealing, as well as the texture or taste. It may seem nonincidental at first, to satisfy a craving with a small piece of chocolate, though because the response to stress is food related, it will continue and become habit forming. The initial sensation to tasting a piece of milk chocolate after handling a difficult client on the job may feel euphoric and then you'll want another piece, followed by another. A pattern emerges that becomes a link between your emotions and food. The portions may also grow, as you soothe your woes, but in the end, there is no solution, and eating habits become difficult to maintain.

How can you avoid the pitfalls of emotional eating? Take into consideration your mood when you reach for the next snack. Where are you currently? At work, home, at an event or in a situation that causes a certain feeling? Most importantly, determine if you are actually hungry, by using the scale between one to ten. If you rate your hunger closer to ten, it may be a good idea to eat, though make sure you find a calm place without stress before you begin your meal. Experiencing hunger means it's a good time to eat, but only with as little pressure and emotional impact as possible. If you are in a busy environment, find another space to decompress and relax. Practice deep breathing and decide where to enjoy your meal.

When you crave food, ask yourself what you are feeling. Are you angry, sad or stressed? If you are experiencing an intense emotion or in a state of frustration, hold off on eating until you can bring yourself into a calm space, away from any surroundings that are contributing to these emotions. It can take less time than you think and can be as easy as leaving the office or workspace and going outdoors to walk in a nearby park. If that option is not available, choose a quiet place in your workplace with minimal distractions. Sometimes this can be difficult to find if your space is very busy and hectic. Even a few moments in a bathroom or an empty room for five minutes can make a big difference. When you feel calmer, you may notice those cravings subside. It's ok if they don't, as stressful situations are not easy to diffuse. A few minutes can make the difference between reacting to your emotions with food and choosing another means to acknowledge and remedy the situation with mediation and a few moments of solitude.

Food is a good distraction. To identify your emotional connection to food means to acknowledge it mindfully, instead of making an excuse for it. It's common and easy to excuse eating simply, to soothe a bad day or situation. Some emotions can be traced back to childhood or a significant experience that triggers a response with food. In these cases, it may take longer to delve deep within our mind to find that reason for the response. Mindfulness helps us by taking a scan of our body and thoughts in that very moment and finding the root of that emotion. Are we feeling a quicker heartbeat or shallow breathing or something in our stomach? If someone upsets or insults you, food can quiet the injury temporarily, but it will only arise later when you realize that that source of conflict and emotion was not handled, but rather, avoided with food.

Pitfalls of Traditional Dieting And How to Avoid It?

Diets don't recognize hunger as the solution but rather the problem: ignore your body and follow the meal plans and restrictions. While many diets currently offer variations and plenty of options, they are very similar in avoiding your body's natural signals and responses to hunger and food. Adherence to diets also work with a reward system of success that does not connect to your emotion and body but rather how many inches or weight you lose. Social media groups often encourage followers to post before and after pictures, which is meant to help other people see results and stick with the diet. Unfortunately, the opposite reaction or result occurs: People may see an unattainable goal or one that takes an awful lot of effort to achieve. Losing weight is only part of the battle, as most people who follow a diet, even if successful, gain all or most of the lost pounds back. Keeping the weight off often means continuing the diet indefinitely, or risk gaining more again. Exercise is also a means to keep up the success of a diet and often seen as a necessary chore, rather than an enjoyment of movement in of itself. This creates a cycle of success and failure, as dieters fall off of the food plan and either overdo the exercise to compensate or fall behind, only to start all over again or quit.

How many diets have you tried? If you attempted one diet, chances are, you have tried several. The first diet is almost never successful in the long run and once this is done, you may stop altogether or start a new one. It's a pattern that many people repeat with the goal of life-long weight loss, maintenance, and good health. Focusing only on the foods we eat, restricting them without paying any attention to what our bodies are telling us, without noticing our emotional state and hunger level is where diets inevitably fail. Intuitive eating establishes a long-term pattern of natural eating habits in tune with our mind and body's signals. By paying attention to our emotions and reactions in the moment, every time we crave food, we will be able to stop the impulsive reaction to eat when we are not hungry and restore and establish a healthy eating pattern that will last a lifetime.

Avoid Extreme Changes to the Way You Eat

We may learn about a new diet, cleansing fast or similar get-thin-fast fad, along with testimonies of how successful it is. This is common for many diets and juice fasts, but they will change over time. Avoid them and focus on what your needs are. If you are tempted to try a diet, realize that it's an emotional response to getting a result quickly. The most popular reason for dieting is weight loss, and there is no one way that fits everyone. Even with success, there is a limit to how long a diet will achieve the result. The ability to measure your body's needs, assess your hunger will be sabotaged with diets that don't connect to your individual requirements, and for this reason, its best to avoid them completely.

Diets cause stress and force us to adhere to a restrictive plan, increasing pressure to see results within a relatively short time frame. It is a culture that has lasted for generations, with each new way of eating promising better results than the last. The way of dieting aims to place you in a box of options, limiting what you can choose, whether it's by portion size, calories, carbohydrates or when we are allowed to eat. If we meet certain milestones, we may feel more motivated to continue, or take a break and "treat" ourselves with a "cheat" meal or similarly restricted food. This will result in increased pressure to jump back into the diet with even more focus and restriction. We ignore the signals our body sends us, such as hunger pangs when we should eat, and feel punished if we don't see results right away.

Chapter 6. The Heaviness of Nonacceptance

Eating to avoid emotion may be a deliberate strategy or a habitual pattern that is almost unconscious. In other words, you may experience an emotion, wish to control it, and, consciously or not, use food to avoid or alter it, implicitly reinforcing the notion that you just can't cope with your feelings.

Experiential avoidance, or attempts to avoid, suppress, or change negative events, including feelings, thoughts, and bodily sensations, underlies both emotional suffering (Hayes et al. 1996) and emotional eating.

Pain is a part of living. We are all faced with difficult emotions, painful memories, and obstacles. Many individuals describe their struggle with emotions as greater than their experience of physical pain. Dissatisfaction with one's shape and size may include a combination of emotional and physical discomfort. How do you cope with uncomfortable thoughts, feelings, and sensations?

Avoidance and control strategies can bring advantages. Our ancestors survived, in part, by taking precautions and gaining some degree of control over their situations. These coping strategies are thus in our DNA, and they are, in themselves, neither good nor bad. They are, however, sometimes ineffective in our daily lives. When are attempts to control our situations effective? If we need to concentrate on an important project, it is effective if we remove distractions. If we want to lose weight, it is useful if we limit the amount of sweets and processed fatty foods in the home. But attempts to control situations often fail, and this usually happens when they are too rigid and/or when we try to use them in situations where they will not work. For example, if you decide to pursue a highly restrictive diet in which you drastically reduce your intake of calories, you are likely to binge at some point because you will feel deprived. Control is also not feasible when we try to radically alter inalterable aspects of the body, such as the aging process. The next exercise is designed to give you some practice discerning when control strategies might be effective and when they might not be.

Exercise: Control or Let Go?

Spend a moment writing about or thinking of three examples of situations where your efforts at control seem not to work.

Taking each situation in turn, think of aspects you can control and aspects you cannot.

For example:

I can't control the fact that I experience food cravings.

I can't control what other people think of me.

I can't totally control how much I enjoy various activities.

I can make sure I purchase only healthy food items for my home, but I cannot control what my family members or guests choose to bring over.

Certain strategies we employ to "fix" our feelings will inevitably cause us to feel them more intensely. Even the proverbial "control freak" will often fail when it comes to managing his emotions—you can organize your closets and subdue your children, but it is a lot harder to suppress your own inner life. Still, most of us try to fix our feelings. Who wants to feel fat, anxious, sad, or lonely? But our best efforts to subdue emotional pain often create additional suffering.

Exercise: Letting Go of Strategies to Avoid

Take a moment to think about ways you have tried to manage your emotions. Have you ever avoided the pain of being alone by keeping the television on, incessantly snacking, or using other avoidance behaviors? List as many strategies as you can that you have used to try to avoid or change your feelings.

What are the feelings you find most challenging to experience?

How might you practice accepting those feelings?

Imagine that you are wearing your favorite pair of suede shoes, and you are walking down the street on your way to an important meeting. Suddenly, it starts to pour. You wait under an awning for several minutes, but wishing the rain away or remaining under the awning will not change the weather. You wait and worry and become physically tense. Your shoes will be ruined! But if you continue to wait and miss your meeting, the lost opportunity may equal the cost of several pairs of shoes.

Trying to control emotions is like trying to keep your shoes dry in a rainstorm. You may try, and certain techniques may even work in the short term—if you are caught in a rainstorm, it may be useful to step inside for some time. But what if you chose to walk—even to dance—in the rain? What if the deluge became part of your day, an anecdote for the meeting, something (among the many things life throws at you) that couldn't stop you?

We can't control our emotions any more than we can control the weather. Let's try this: Get really happy right now. Tough, isn't it? Try harder! What do you notice? Joy, sadness, confusion, loss—none of these can be turned on or off at our command. Willpower is simply not helpful here. In fact, efforts to switch melancholy into the "all joy, all the time" channel will generally magnify your sadness into real misery. Why set yourself up? Why "fail" at something that is not possible?

Mark's Story

Mark was diagnosed with attention deficit disorder (ADD) as a child. Understandably, he still struggles with organization and concentration. Mark works in sales, and given his ADD, he has strategically developed a plan to overprepare for meetings, thoroughly considering any potential obstacles.

One day on the way to a high-stakes meeting, Mark began to sweat. He tried to force himself to stop sweating by thinking about how humiliating it would be to be visibly dripping in front of his colleagues. This only led to more sweating. Worse, Mark felt so uncomfortable and anxious that he actually bought himself a large cold beer and a cheeseburger, despite the facts that he was on his way to a business meeting and has high cholesterol. Mark's efforts to manage his anxiety and control his body were backfiring, and it wasn't the first time. He had a very well-conceived plan in place to handle meetings, but he still felt exhausted before and after important meetings. He increasingly tried to soothe himself with comfort foods, television, and alcohol. As you can imagine, the more effort he invested in controlling his body and avoiding his anxiety, the more anxious he actually felt and the less efficient he was in his work. And on the day I've just described, the more he sweated emotionally, the more he sweated physically—a strong metaphor for how ineffectual our attempts to control the uncontrollable can be.

Hiding Feelings Causes You to Feel More

While you may inhibit the ways you express an emotion, physiologically you experience increased sensations in parallel with any attempt to suppress your emotions (Gross and Levenson 1997). For example, if you try to avoid feeling anxious, you may reduce the look of panic on your face to some degree, but your heart rate will increase as a result of your trying to fake calmness. So inhibiting your expression of negative emotions does not provide relief from your experience of the feeling, but does the opposite. Researchers (e.g., Wegner, Quillian, and Houston 1996) also suspect that trying to inhibit emotions limits your ability to organize information. Think about it: if you're focused on managing your expression, it's difficult to concentrate on and attend to what's happening around you. In Mark's situation, he may sometimes be so attuned to his attempt to appear calm that he fails to notice how engaged his colleagues are with his presentation. Suppressing emotions may also affect your relationships with others. If you rigidly control your expression, will people in your life be aware of your struggle? And with your attention absorbed in managing how you appear, will you have much of a chance of seeing what is happening with them? Not likely, and the combined result is that you will probably feel more and more isolated and less likely to elicit or express supportive and loving behavior.

Feel Less, Eat More?

How does suppressing emotion lead to increased eating of comfort foods? One possibility is that the act of suppression is itself emotionally depleting. You may be expending energy on stifling your feelings, leaving you with few resources when it comes to monitoring food (Vohs and Heatherton 2000). Interestingly, if you are not on a diet, you are less likely to indulge, as there is less pressure surrounding food choices.

So here is the sequence: You start feeling sad. You don't express the emotion, but try to stop feeling it. You now have less control when it comes to choosing what you eat and are more likely to eat unhealthy comfort foods. Then, you feel guilt when you do turn to comfort foods—another negative emotion! Any bets on what happens when you suppress the guilt? When you maintain rigid standards of perfection, or are not willing to accept yourself as you are, food serves as a temporary escape (Heatherton and Baumeister 1991), but escaping once makes it that much more likely you'll be driven to seek escape again, and again, forgetting that this strategy doesn't actually work in the long term.

So what might happen if you didn't need to escape yourself with food? What might happen if you compassionately acknowledged and addressed your sadness?

Chapter 7. Important Things to Know About Your Emotional Brain

It is a Powerful Rapid-Response System

The emotional brain is first in line after the brainstem to receive most incoming sensory information. Since it's adapted to dealing with spontaneous life-or-death challenges in an unforgiving environment, its reaction speed is far greater than that of the cortex.

Because it is more essential to immediate survival, it has the power to override the cortex altogether if it is triggered enough. In situations where pausing to think could be what gets you killed, this is a good thing. A practical consideration here is that the emotional brain can begin to react to incoming information and lock out the cortex before the cortex even has a chance to get in the game.

Being confronted with highly appealing food is not a life-or-death event, but it can cause intense reactivity in the emotional system just the same. Anything that triggers the emotional brain—the sight, smell, mention, or mere thought of certain foods—can activate the mechanisms that begin to lock out the cortex.

For successful food management in the modern world, you must minimize those circumstances in which your emotional brain can start to spin up and take over before your cortex can save the day.

It Prioritizes the Present

Life in the wild is all about surviving the moment and helping one's offspring to do the same, so the emotional brain is anchored in the present. It does not readily learn from delayed consequences nor does it readily embrace delayed gratification; these inputs are too far removed in time to motivate it to a meaningful degree.

It reacts the most to whatever is most immediate, which is why you're drawn so powerfully to a trigger food rather than to the less tangible results of the more distant future. The tortured debate in your head might sound like, This is going to be so great—I can't wait! vs., I always end up hating myself after I eat like this. Why isn't that enough to make me stop wanting to do it??

It's worth noting that while the emotional brain is not motivated by future results, it is the emotional brain that will experience them when the time comes. That's where you experience the suffering created by short-sighted, impulsive choices.

It is also where you bask in victory and contentment when things turn out well.

Because of the limitations described above, though, the emotional brain can't prioritize future results when making decisions; in a way, it can't see where it's going. Only the cortex can fully comprehend the future, so only the cortex can determine which choices will make the emotional brain the happiest both now and in the future.

It Develops Strong Biases

When you have found something enjoyable, that item or experience gets filed in the "like it and want more of it" category, perhaps intensely so. You'll give that experience the benefit of the doubt going forward, classifying it as a good thing because you enjoyed it in the past.

Because it's nice to figure something out and not have to decide about it again, you'll want to keep that mindset. You will, therefore, tend to minimize, rationalize, deny, or simply ignore new evidence that contradicts your initial evaluation.

Consider what happens once you've identified a favorite food, for example. Let's say this food makes you all happy just thinking about it, and you get it as much as you possibly can. Now you find out that this favorite food has some ingredients you find worrisome. Logically, you'd walk away, but this isn't logical. You love the food, so you reassure yourself with rationalizations like, "They wouldn't sell it if it was bad for us," or "I eat a lot of other things that are healthier so it all balances out," or "This is just normal--everybody eats this."

If you heard about the same questionable ingredients in a food you hadn't yet tried, you might feel just fine passing it up. Since it's a food you already love, however, the mental contortions begin. You keep the food in your life and just try a little harder not to think about it. Feelings overpower facts.[1]

How about when you begin to notice that whenever you have certain much-loved foods, you usually end up stuffed, miserable, and hating yourself afterward? Logically, you'd easily walk away from anything that predictably makes you feel miserable and loathsome. Who wouldn't? In this case, you wouldn't. Your emotional brain has fixated on these foods as something it wants, based strictly on how enjoyable you hope the foods will be while you're eating them. You'll be hard pressed to come up with enough evidence to get your emotional brain to reconsider this position because again, feelings overpower facts.

The emotional brain's tendency to adopt stubborn biases shows up in many ways above and beyond food issues.[2] Addiction, for example, has to do in part with the emotional brain categorizing something as very desirable, then doggedly pursuing it even in the absence of the expected reward. In other words, you're doing something that's not giving you all you were hoping for, but you feel compelled to keep at it because it really seems like the reward should come if you just try hard enough.

The emotional brain will cling to an established bias like this in the face of many, many experiences that fail to bear it out. The tendency is to keep believing rather than destroying that particular mental structure and building something new. This is why we keep turning to food despite ourselves.

Phobias, on the other hand, are in part about the emotional brain categorizing something as a threat, and then doggedly avoiding it even in the absence of the expected harm. The emotional brain will cling to the fear despite things repeatedly turning out just fine, as feelings overrule facts yet again.

Aversions are far less intense than phobias, but can be another example of the emotional brain categorizing something negatively despite information that suggests otherwise.

Many people feel resistant to the idea of nutritious food and regular exercise, for instance, despite the fact that both routinely create enjoyable results. In this case, the emotional brain is convinced that these practices are burdensome rather than rewarding simply because the rewards don't come quickly enough and worse, because some effort is required up front. The emotional brain maintains this bias despite experience to the contrary that with just a little more time, these choices create much more happiness and satisfaction than do most other alternatives.

It Has a Long Memory

The emotional brain usually prefers the familiar—"the devil you know"—to the unknown, even if the familiar has obvious drawbacks. This is why you may feel resistant to trying healthier patterns even though you know you need them—you resist them because they are different. It is also why you may abandon those patterns at some future point even if they've been working well for you—some part of you yearns to just relax back into the familiar, despite the fact that it caused the problems that spurred you into change in the first place. A brief glimpse into nervous system function will explain why we have these tendencies.

Whenever you think or do anything, it is made possible by the transmission of electrical signals in your nervous system. These signals move from one nerve cell (neuron) to the next, activating the bodily systems necessary to execute whatever action you have decided to take.

Much like a footpath in the woods that becomes easier to find with repeated use, neural pathways become more robust with practice.[3] The stronger the neural pathway, the more easily and efficiently you can perform that particular action. This is why practice makes perfect, but it's also why old habits die hard.

Your overeating patterns have been practiced thousands of times over many years, creating neural superhighways to enable their operation.

When you go on to create new neural pathways for more fulfilling patterns, the old pathways fall into disuse, but don't disappear. The old pathways remain—well-built but inactive— right alongside the newer ones which support better outcomes, but which are still under construction.

In day-to-day life, this means that when you stop intentionally choosing the newer path, you'll automatically default back to the old one that you know so well.

You can do this so smoothly that you don't even realize it, perhaps "finding" yourself doing something like eating out of a bag of cookies, pulling up to a drive-through, or finishing the kids' leftovers. The shift into the old pattern can be that seamless, and it happens in an instant.

You may dream of a time when you can completely forget about the old, painful days of the addiction but the truth is that the neural pathways for it will always remain in place. This is why the risk of relapse generally lasts to some degree for a lifetime. You should exercise extreme caution whenever you notice yourself thinking something like, I should be able to do this safely now.

This is not to say that all you have to look forward to is struggling through the remainder of your life, one white-knuckled day at a time. Those new neural pathways, if you've built them to the right places, will actually enable you to calm down and enjoy your life more than ever before.

Nor is it the case that perfect performance is necessary for you to succeed. Momentary lapses are to be expected, but should also be taken seriously. A lapse—any behavior that you didn't plan on, couldn't control, or ultimately made you at all unhappy—is a serious warning that if you're not more cautious going forward, things are likely to get worse.

A lapse with food compares to driving a car and wandering out of your lane until you hit the rumble strips along the edge. Nothing truly bad happens, but you've been put on notice that disaster got closer than usual. Ignore the warning at your own risk.

You're likely to have lapses—hopefully, mostly small ones—for the rest of your life. Just heed them as the warning signs that they are and learn as much as you can from them. Properly examined, each one makes you stronger. Over time, you'll have them less often and recover from them more quickly, but odds are that they'll still pop up periodically. The best response is to just keep learning and moving forward.

It is Poorly Matched to Today's World

There is a profound difference between what enhances survival in the wild and what enhances it in modern life. As a result, our wellbeing is now threatened by the same behavioral tendencies that have protected us for most of our history.

Our preference for sweets is a perfect example—it works out well in the wild, leading us to essential nutrients. In the modern world, however, that same taste preference leads us to overindulgence in products that accelerate numerous disease and addictive processes.

The dilemma is how to channel the power of the emotional brain so that it can once again drive positive outcomes rather than harmful ones, despite being in an unnatural environment that constantly supplies it with misinformation.

This is an easier task to face when you remember what the emotional brain does for you, despite its unique quirks and vulnerabilities.

It is Still Why Life is Worth Living

Have you ever loved someone or felt the warmth of knowing someone loves you? Do you have a hobby or interest that you look forward to doing, which engages you so much that you lose track of time while you're doing it? Have you ever felt the thrill of an unexpected and wonderful surprise? Have you ever felt an upwelling of confidence from overcoming a challenge you weren't sure you could manage? Have you ever had a moment which felt absolutely perfect?

These experiences and all like them come to you courtesy of your emotional brain, because it is where your feelings develop. It's not simply a source of joy and happiness, of course; all of the pain in life happens there too, including the guilt, shame and regret of uncontrolled overeating.

Many people, upon learning that a specific part of the brain drives their compulsive eating, express an urgent desire to have that part surgically removed. Even if that were possible, it would mean that you'd never again have any of the feelings that make for a fully dimensional life. Imagine a life in which everything feels like nothing—do you really want that?

The task, then, is to appreciate what your emotional brain makes possible for you while learning to use it and take care of it more effectively, based on the somewhat odd requirements of today's world. When you do, you'll find that your emotional brain will be the source of more peace, joy, and true contentment than ever before.

Unexpected Hazards of Modern Life

Modern life offers an abundance of opportunities of many kinds, which actually poses a serious challenge to the emotional brain. When you understand how this works, you can set up your life to be much simpler, calmer, more satisfying, and more enjoyable.

The Problem of Too Much

The emotional brain is geared toward rapid judgement of the elements in its world, and rapid action based on that judgement. In a world of scarce resources and limited opportunities, the "get what you can whenever you can get it" system works well. There is little need for behavioral self-regulation in nature simply because there is so little opportunity for excess of any kind.

This is not to say we are incapable of self-regulation. The problem is that our capacity for it does not reside in the emotional brain, which happens to have the greatest immediate power in how decisions get made.

Most of us now have constant access to hyper palatable food. The emotional brain reacts to this abundance just as it would to the limited opportunities for which it is adapted: by trying to have it all. It is very unnatural to have food available and have the physical ability to eat more of it, yet choose to stop eating. The emotional brain simply does not operate this way.

Food is not the only field on which this problem plays out. Given the emotional brain's preference for quick reward and for exploiting immediate opportunities in general, it's not hard to see how abundance and easy opportunity of any kind has the potential to take a wrong turn.

Consider some other everyday indulgences that carry a known risk of addiction: alcohol use, drug use, smoking, sex, spending, gambling, and online activities. It's certainly possible to pursue any of these without lapsing into self-destructiveness and many people do, but a great many also fail in the attempt. Loss of personal control in such instances shows you an emotional brain unintentionally self-destructing as it applies the "get all you can" strategy to a situation in which it is possible to get too much. "Enough" is not an emotional brain concept. The emotional brain, left to its own devices, is unable to stop until the negative consequences of excess make it too painful to continue, or until there is simply no more opportunity.

The Powerful, Defenseless Emotional Brain

The cortex can easily provide the self-regulation that makes it possible for the emotional brain to live happily and healthily in a world of too much.

The problem is that the emotional brain is intensely activated by opportunity, and can be triggered into an internal power grab that locks out the cortex. If this happens, the emotional brain is left unguided where it can't protect itself. Chaos, frustration, and regret are the predictable result.

The need for frequent, deliberate self-management is quite new to us as a species, yet its importance is intensifying more with each passing year. The requirement for it now is dramatically higher than it was just 40 to 50 years ago, let alone for all of human history prior to that. It is perhaps understandable that it's been hard for most of us to keep up with what it takes to survive in our very different world of the present.

At the time of this writing, reality TV is a well-established genre, including a subset devoted to survival in the wild with minimal support. These programs show how valuable our basic drives still are once we're back in a setting that fits them. Cast members do exactly what we all want to do: they eat everything they can find and rest whenever they can. Their setting involves few opportunities for food and rest, so this promotes survival.

In our setting with endless opportunity for both, the same choices are ruining millions of lives.

Self-Management for Life

It is vital to understand the mismatch between how our brains work and what is required by the conditions in which we now live. Our core survival drives, left unchecked in conditions of overabundance, result in behavior that promotes self-destruction rather than survival.

We are well-equipped to handle this mismatch as long as we can keep the cortex engaged. So, how can we do that? The answer is not in strengthening the cortex so that it can get better at controlling the impulsive emotional brain, because that isn't possible.

What does work is to keep the emotional brain calm enough to be receptive to higher-level strategies. It is when the emotional brain becomes reactive—as with excitement, anticipation, depression, anxiety, or anger—that it can start to override the cortex. This is why no amount of logic seems sufficient to overcome an intense desire to eat.

As long as you continue to live in an environment of easy excess, it will be necessary to remain conscious and intentional about food in your life. This is not a punishment or a burden—it is simply a factual requirement of how we now live. Your emotional brain will always be on hot standby, ready to spring into action with those old drives if it is triggered too much. The only solution is to minimize how much that happens.

Overcoming the Diet Mentality

This book espouses a non-diet approach to weight management that flies in the face of our conditioning. Dieting seems to be embedded in our culture to the point of being compulsory. Do you remember the time when you simply ate when you were hungry and didn't worry about calories, weight, health, or how you looked? If you're like me, that was many years ago. And, it's not our fault. There are many forces conspiring to keep us unhappy and dissatisfied with the way we look and the way we eat. One of the biggest forces is the hundreds of diets vying for our attention and our money.

Review your dieting history. How many have you been on? Are you on one now? The research I conducted revealed that participants were actively on a diet for an average of 39 percent of their lives—some starting their diets as young as five years old! And, the negative impact from this early indoctrination to dieting ranges from being overweight to feeling miserable about ourselves.

Diets Don't Work

It is easy to be attracted by promises of amazing results in thirty days, the diet that a friend is trying, or a claim that you'll be smarter, stronger, and happier with a particular product. You intuitively know the results you seek are going to take some time and effort, but you still hold out hope for the quick fix. The secret hope is you will melt down to your perfect shape or have a healthier body and it's all going to happen quickly and easily. But, let's be honest with each other. If any of the diets you've been on had been successful (however you define that), would you really be reading this book?

Diets, in particular, have done very little to help people lose weight or curb anyone's appetite. At least that's what the statistics say. America's obesity rates are among the highest in the world. Millions of people are on diets, yet two thirds of US adults are overweight or obese and these numbers and waistlines are continuing to grow (Ogden et al. 2014). There is a multibillion dollar global weight-loss industry banking on the fact that you'll need its diet products for a long time.

Researchers at the University of California, Los Angeles analyzed the results from thirty-one long-term studies of diets and concluded that even if dieters lose weight initially, the majority of people on diets gain all of the weight back, plus more. "Yo-yo" dieters, people who lose and gain weight, especially repeatedly, actually increase their risks for diabetes, hypertension, heart disease, and metabolic syndrome (Mann et al. 2007). This review of the literature demonstrates that you are actually better off never having gone on a diet in the first place.

I've heard plenty of anecdotal evidence of dismal dieting failures. Stacey, a long-term dieter, stated, "I have done so many diets since I was fifteen years old, I can tell you how many calories are in any kind of food." She went on to validate what the research tells us: "Diets never worked out. No matter what kind of diet plan I have ever tried, nothing was permanent. I would weigh myself constantly, and the weight always came back."

Like Stacey, many dieters are frustrated and have thrown up their hands in disgust. Paula said, "Because of my diet history, I have reached a point where I do not even feel capable of dieting. All the platitudes in the world cannot motivate me at this point.

I have tried just about every diet possible and that is not a way for me to live. I am one of those people that hear the word 'diet' and immediately start eating everything in sight."

Even if you are someone who says you don't diet, you might be surprised at how influenced you are by the diet mentality. You say you aren't on a diet, but you secretly dread the times when your food options are not within your control, you examine food carefully before you eat it, you label foods as "good" and "bad," or you have a lot of shoulds and shouldn'ts when it comes to eating. You may say you just want to eat healthily, but you deny yourself the pleasure of eating if it doesn't fall into the "good" category. (Note: There is a difference between the diet mentality and mindfully deciding you don't want to eat certain foods after an examination of their taste and effect on your body.) Because of their omnipresence, dieting thoughts and images are ingrained in us all.

Take a moment right now and check in with yourself. Even though this book takes a clearly "non-diet" approach, you might unconsciously be hoping it's the next new diet plan that will actually work. Be honest with yourself. The "dieting mind" is very clever.

Why Diets Don't Work

So, why don't diets work? First, diets overly restrict the kinds of food or how much food you can eat, so you would never be able to continue to eat this way in the long term. Eating a limited variety of food or consuming deathly low calorie counts will help you lose weight while you're on the diet, but when you go off of it and start eating as you normally do (which you will), you gain the weight back.

Third, what happens when you tell yourself you can't have something to eat? You want it! Right? And when you finally have it, you'll have a lot of it. Oftentimes you'll eat your forbidden food alone and in secret while no one is watching. You'll gobble it down as fast as you can so nobody sees you. You'll have to have a lot of it because you tell yourself you're never going to have it again.

My friend Lynn wouldn't allow herself to have candy and sweets at home, so she would steal those goodies from the desk drawers of her coworkers. Of course, it was kind of a joke because all of her coworkers knew she was doing it. They gladly stocked their drawers for her stealing pleasure. Janice, a twenty-five-year-old athlete, would only sneak cookies and sweets at work because her athletic husband tried to keep her on a very strict calorie and carb count. Both of these women were not going to be denied, but they didn't really get to enjoy their treats, indulging alone and in secret.

Fourth, when you're relying solely on an outside source (such as a diet) to tell you what to eat, you're not paying attention to the wisdom of your own body. Until you begin to listen to and trust your inner wisdom (instead of a diet) about what, when, why, and how much you eat, it is unlikely you will be able to change the way you eat. The body has amazing sensors for what food is healthy, what food is poison to the system, how much food it needs to consume, and what nutrition it needs. Animals in the wild live and eat by instinctive internal wisdom and forage the fields and forests for the food that will meet their nutritional requirements. No one had to give them a nutrition class, and yet they are very capable of knowing what to eat. We are no less intuitive than animals, but most humans have cut themselves off from the body's natural guidance.

This brings me to the last and maybe most important point: diets tend to take the joy out of food. On a diet, the only joy is found when you cheat—and you will! My philosophy is that food is a wonderful part of our lives, to be enjoyed and savored. A non-diet approach to weight management is one that celebrates the pleasure found in culinary delights of all kinds. When you truly savor your food, you are slowing down to taste the moment and the juiciness of life.

Beginning Steps to Take

Under your nose, in your belly, on your tongue, in your eyes, and in your mind you have the knowledge you need to be wisely instructed about what, when, why, and how much to eat. Instead of eating to fix or deny your feelings, you will learn to respond to difficult times with kindness and courage. You will uncover the thoughts and beliefs that keep sabotaging your efforts to eat better and be healthier so that YOU are in the driver's seat when you make decisions about how to eat and live. Along with the transformation in how you relate to food, you can discover an admiration for your body (no matter what size you are) that supports your efforts to take better care of it.

Before you go any farther, here are a few things I'd like you to consider that will help you turn your focus inward.

1. Get Off the Diets

If you aren't on one, great. Only by not dieting can you give yourself a chance to discover your internal sources of guidance.

However, if your doctor has you on a specific regimen for a medical issue, by all means continue on it. The skills you learn will help you feel better about, succeed at, and enjoy the diet that you need to be on.

2. Get Off the Scale

Despite any slight to significant anxiety this creates for you, I hope you give yourself the opportunity to discover what staying off the scale can teach you. Not relying on an external measurement to monitor your weight helps you begin your journey inward. This is the first step toward listening to your internal signals to guide how you eat. Besides, you can gauge getting heavier or lighter by paying attention to how your body looks and feels or how tight or loose your pants fit.

Has getting on the scale ever helped you lose weight? Or are you ever happy with the number on the scale? I've asked these questions to many people and the answer is usually a resounding no. Getting off the scale lets you stop creating one time a day that you purposely feel disappointed with yourself.

Personally, my game with the scale was to set a weight that I wanted to but couldn't realistically meet. Years went by and then a miracle happened. I finally, and incredibly, reached my goal. I was so happy—for about two seconds (literally)—before I decided I needed to be five pounds lighter! A long time ago, I left the scale with my ex-husband, and I've been a lot happier ever since.

One issue that makes not weighing yourself difficult is a trip to the doctor, since the first thing you are asked to do is get on the scale. Having dealt with this for years, here is what I suggest: tell the nurse you will get on the scale but you don't want to know how much you weigh. Even if you look, oftentimes the weight is in kilograms. Unless you're better than me at converting kilograms into pounds, you won't know your weight anyway. I admit I've even been a bit of a rebel in the past and just declined to get on the scale, but I've been informed by a doctor that recording your weight at each visit is required by insurance and

Medicaid. It's probably better to be friendly and let them weigh you.

3. Set One Goal (Besides Weight Loss) to Get You Started

However, for the time being I would like you to take the focus off of a number on the scale. A number is only an external validation of who you are and how you want to feel. So, I'd like to encourage you to go a little upstream from the goal of weight loss. In other words, how would you like to be acting or thinking differently that would ultimately result in you losing weight?

Take a moment to stop and close your eyes while you take a couple of deep breaths. See what answers arise. Some answers I often hear are "I'd like to eat slower," "I'd like to stop eating before I'm full," "I'd like to stop eating in front of the computer and while I'm reading," and "I'd like to stop eating the last bites of food on my children's plates."

If nothing occurred to you this time, keep checking in as you continue reading.

Developing Realistic Confidence

Now! Drum roll, please, for the question every motivation-eliciting pep talk includes: what is the difference between those who succeed in accomplishing a goal, such as urge surfing, and those who do not? I don't want to presume I have the answer to this complex question. So let's slow down and wonder together: What thwarts action? What would potential remedies include?

Imagine that one of your long-standing goals is to run a marathon, twenty-six miles. What steps are necessary to get to the physical fitness level you need to achieve before you can run a marathon? According to Olympic athlete and running coach Jeff Galloway, to prep for the marathon, you begin by running or walking for thirty minutes, twice a week, and you methodically build your endurance over time. In twenty-nine weeks, you can go from being unable to run more than three miles to running twenty-six miles. This is not a late-night infomercial; this is a program thousands of people like you and me have followed to make marathon running a realistic ambition. In order to build a sense of realistic confidence in a goal, then, break a task into manageable chunks. To develop a sense of confidence more generally, regularly challenge yourself.

We are all faced with challenges. Mastery means doing things that make you feel competent and confident (e.g., Linehan 1993b). Self-efficacy, or your beliefs about your ability, has a major impact on your life. You build your sense of self-efficacy through mastery. Some people wait until they feel confident to begin a challenge. What is the alternative? Build competence by deliberately identifying goals that are both difficult and possible. Ask yourself, "Where is my goal on the continuum from effortless to unattainable?" Mastery is all about being in the middle of that spectrum.

Almost any effective program in which you change an existing behavior includes some reasonable step to engender hope to take the next. Think about Alcoholics Anonymous, whose motto is "One day at a time," not "Don't drink for the rest of your life." Chances are the latter sentiment would breed anxiety and thus perhaps lead to drinking, while the former seems manageable and increases the chances of abstinence. A patient of mine once described developing mastery as "tricking the brain" by circumventing paths that lead to resistance. I see taking workable steps as the only way to build optimism, adequately preparing you for change in the relationship between your emotions and food.

Mastery and Urge Surfing

Urge surfing requires a sense of mastery, and surfing urges builds mastery. Knowing you have trained enough that you can run a marathon provides a base of realistic confidence in other areas: "Of course I can ride the urge to order nachos; I've ridden many urges to quit running!" Similarly, repeatedly surfing the urge to order nachos may also establish both a general sense of self-confidence and the confidence that you can resist the next food pitfall.

When your mind sends you the message "Give up! Why bother?" you can thank your mind for that thought. Thanking your mind for a thought is observing the thought without judgment, rather than responding to the thought as though it is a factual alarm. Then, you can cheer yourself on by reminding yourself of difficult urges you've experienced and surfed. Similarly, practicing urge surfing builds mastery. By repeatedly noticing, labeling, and riding urges, you will build your sense of confidence in your ability to give yourself more space between urge and action.

Many people who struggle with eating problems make eating the focus of living. You may feel like you've worked really hard to abstain from emotional eating. Perhaps stepping back and noticing how you excel in other areas will engender renewed realistic confidence that you can end your emotional eating. We have little incentive to pursue goals if we don't have a sense we will accomplish them.

Building mastery in various areas of your life may reduce your vulnerability to intense emotions and urges. Let's say your desire to offer the wittiest toast at your brother's wedding is creating a lot of stress. Taking a course on public speaking with the goal of mastering your public speaking skills and conquering your fear may reduce the anxiety you experience. In addition, when you problem solve and take steps to build your confidence, you may be less likely to turn to food to cope with your nerves about the speech. And knowing you can sit with discomfort (for example, surfing the urge to feign laryngitis to avoid giving the toast) may spill over and influence your sense of mastery to sit with the urge to eat.

Pain with a Purpose

Building mastery muscles requires resistance training. Let's be frank. Running to increase your mileage each week is (literally) no walk in the park. Instant gratification is not the game here (nor will it take you far). Mastery, by definition, will not be instantaneous.

In the short term, mastery requires perseverance. In the long run, mastery will improve your mood and reduce your vulnerability to negative emotions. Over time, engaging in challenging actions purposefully will improve self-esteem and reduce feelings of depression. People often describe feeling more joy from accomplishment than from seeking instant pleasure. You may be struggling with low self-esteem, questioning your ability to experience a sense of accomplishment, and eating to manage your nerves. That is, you may change the way you feel by doing. When thoughts attempt to convince you not to bother with surfing your urges, dealing with your emotions differently, or improving your musical abilities, notice those thoughts—and let them go by like so much background noise. By changing your actual behaviors, you will get unstuck. Eventually, the raucous dissonance in your mind may begin to quiet. Ultimately, you run the marathon with your legs and not your thoughts. It would be nice if your mind helped you along the way, but it is not required. Would you be willing to move your body toward what matters deeply and bring your attention there?

Individuals may travel to a Zen ashram to develop spiritually. They meditate. They also sweep floors. You spend money, travel to a hillside, sit in silence, and scrub toilets. A couple of years ago, I had the opportunity to participate in a meditation retreat with Marsha Linehan, the psychologist who created DBT, in Tucson, Arizona. I envisioned relaxing in the sun, savoring the vegetarian meals, cultivating mindfulness, and becoming a more patient person in a mere five days. I did not expect a 5:30 a.m. wake-up, sitting for six hours a day facing a white wall, and sweeping. All these tasks required mental mastery. After a day of staring at the wall, I broke the practice of silence and asked Marsha if it would be possible to sit outside facing the cacti. She said something along the lines of "Life is about what happens when you're faced with white walls." Anticipating only pleasure, or at least pain-free steps toward growth, may hinder our progress. Thus, the chores we face along the way may be therapeutic. Room service and a concierge will not change your mood in the same way accomplishments change your experience and your sense of self.

The Motivation Myth

"You cannot urge surf or train for the marathon until you are motivated." That statement is a common myth. Motivation is like winning the lottery; it is tenuous and is no guarantee for an enriching life. You are probably thinking you know yourself and you work only when motivated. Do you go to work or do your laundry? Do you feel motivated to do those tasks on a regular basis? Often, even when we experience a surge of motivation, the inspiration is fleeting. Waiting to feel different than you do will mean waiting a long time. Deliberately acting, again and again, will lead to mastery.

Let's get this straight:

1.   Motivation is not a prerequisite for action.

2.   Action leads to action.

3.   Motivation would be nice.

Exercise: Developing Mastery Step by Step

1.   Plan to do at least one thing each day to build a sense of accomplishment. You may practice meditation, take a new

dance class, read a classic you've started and stopped since college, or urge surf.

2.	While engaging in mastery muscle building, be mindful. Notice what you are doing and stay in the moment with it. Mile three is simply (and perfectly) mile three, not a countdown to mile twenty-six. You don't need to analyze your performance. Let go of judgments. This is a time to increase your range of what you believe is possible. Cheer yourself on.

3.	Gradually increase the difficulty of the goal you pursue over time.

Practicing Nonjudgmental Mastery

Nonjudgmental mastery may sound like a paradox—how are you aware of advancing and becoming increasingly competent if you don't judge? Similarly, not judging urges may seem counterintuitive. Well, facts are the antithesis of judgment. "I ran five miles this week and last week I ran four miles" is not a judgment, it's a matter of fact. Observing, "I sat with my emotions," is also a statement of fact. Describing facts is not judging, and it can be free of the psychological side effects of judging. When you label yourself as having had a "bad" run, how likely are you to either return to the track or notice your mood improve? Similarly, labeling urges as "bad" will increase your struggle. However, considering, "Is engaging in this urge effective?" may facilitate positive action.

Mastery is not achieved to get rid of a negative emotional state or prevent a new one. Trying to force yourself to feel other than you do will maintain feeling X and add feeling Y. You feel sad and you work on a New York Times crossword puzzle, wishing you could feel better, and then you feel sad and frustrated. The alternative is noticing you feel sad, accepting the feeling, and fully engaging in the crossword puzzle for the sake of mastery, not to minimize your sadness.

Chapter 8. Sustainable Ways To Practice Intuitive Eating

After seeing how effective intuitive eating is in maintaining optimal weight and overall good health, chances are you will wish to embark on it forthwith. While that is what we wish for, it is important to be aware that there is no journey devoid of challenges. For instance, you may have people close to you pressing you to join them in their weight loss program. While you do not want to sound haughty, you need to learn to be firm about the journey to good health that you want to take. You need to be able to tell your friends and colleagues you appreciate the need to cut excess weight, but you have discovered a better way; a stress-free way. They may actually wish to join you instead.

Nevertheless, you could still face your personal demons, and these you need to have a way of tackling.

Here below are some ways to ensure you remain steadfast on the road of intuitive eating:

1.Practice Hara hachi bu

What, for the sake of healthy eating, is that? Well, it is a saying from the Okinawans of Japan that relates to how you should gauge when to stop eating. What the Okinawans generally mean by that saying is that you need to stop eating when you are 80% full. It is that 20 minute disconnect between your mouth and your stomach that the Okinawa principle seems to tie to.

It is thought that this mindset by the Okinawas has had an impact on their health, as they are said to be the healthiest group of people on earth. Attaining the age of 100yrs is no big deal for an Okinawa. In fact, the average man on the island lives to be 78yrs while the average woman goes up to 86yrs. The point here is: eat enough, not too much. Get satisfied, but not stuffed.

2.Do not categorize food as either good or bad

After all, isn't there a saying that too much of whatever it is can be poisonous? The wise have it, the Bible has it, and even professional psychologists back it up. Avoid going all out to look for specific foods because they are the ones you deem good, and having such a bad attitude towards certain foods just because you deem them bad that you almost develop goose pimples when you see them. That can be really stressful. And what does stress do? The cortisol and its weight-gain catalyzing role takes over, anxiety builds, and you get distracted from the main goal of listening to your body.

Please note that nobody is advocating recklessness. For instance, it is common knowledge that fibrous foods or whole foods are biologically beneficial to the body and we cannot alter biology. They help the body keep blood sugar at the right levels and the liver working optimally. So, yes, go for them.

All successful intuitive eaters do is to emancipate themselves from being too particular about the food they feed their bodies. The strict dieters take time to distinguish sources of fiber, often categorizing arrow roots and sweet potatoes as bad because they are carbohydrates. Intuitive eaters say, this is unprocessed food and my body desires it – on with it. And that way you will enjoy your freedom, your palate will feel good, and your body will not have cravings. Thus, your stomach and your taste buds will find a common balance, the result of which will be a happy, healthy you.

3.Identify hobbies and practice them

An idle mind, someone said, is the devil's workshop. In our case, the devil is the urge to eat simply to pass time. In fact, it is when you are idling – not resting but really idle – that you begin to analyze how many things are not going right in your life. As if anyone's life was perfect! And once the negatives begin flowing, the nearest consolation is food. Remember no matter how nutritious the food is, if your body does not require it when you eat it, you will be messing up your health.

That is why you need to find something to do to keep you from emotional eating. How about taking a walk and taking in nature's beauty? Not only is it healthy in terms of breathing fresh air, but a bit of exercise is always welcome. After all, intuitive eating does not preclude you from doing other healthy things like exercising and keeping the company of positive thinking friends.

4.Be real with your distractions

Whoever said something about serving two masters was right. You are bound to upset one. In our case, the ideal environment for intuitive eating is one where the TV is switched off and you do not have your laptop open before you. Even going through your phone messages as you eat is no good.

Did we speak of getting attuned to your body? You can only do that when your full attention is on it. It will, then, be very easy for you to register the signs of satiety and to stop right where the Okinawas would. And when your mind has finally registered the total amount of food that has gone into your stomach, it will not tell your tummy it has been overstuffed; rather it will give approval and tell it – you are no longer hungry.

On the overall, it is the freedom that comes with intuitive eating that becomes your redeemer. You will know you are on the right track when you no longer wince when someone hands you junk food at a party, or when you do not despise your friends for eating unhealthy snacks in your presence. After all, you will be in control, and you will not feel like partaking unless your body wants the food. Your appetite will be whetted by the state of your body and mind, and not by what the eyes see.

Chapter 9. Hands-On Strategies to Prevent and Overcome Binge Eating

If you struggle with binge eating, you know how easy it is to turn to food whenever there is a problem in life. Rather than pack on the calories and unwanted pounds, here are some hands-on behavioral strategies to help break the cycle of binge eating.

Managing Stress

Stress is one of the major trigger factors for binge eaters. When the going gets tough, it's easy to turn to that refrigerator or take a spin through the drive through to make a big order of fast food. Rather than make food the solution the next time life's burdens are wearing you down, find other outlets for your stress. Exercise is one of the best alternatives, keeping you occupied and helping you to stay in shape as well. You can establish a regular routine that will relieve pressure on a daily basis. Consider going to a massage therapist or taking up yoga to break the stranglehold of tension in your life. You can find a release in many alternatives besides food.

Clean Out the Cabinets

Go through your kitchen and get rid of anything that will tempt you to go on another binge. Ban junk food and sweets in your home. Find healthy substitutes that will not get you in trouble the next time you have cravings and need to satiate your hunger. Stash bags of veggies in the fridge that have already been sliced for snacking. Stock up on fruits. Keep a jug of ice water on hand and have a tall drink any time you are thinking about splurging on snacks. It will help you to feel full and keep on track.

Learn Portion Control

Control your portions to avoid a calorie overload at any meal. One simple trick is to use a saucer at each meal. Only eat what will fit on the plate. You can also try eating several, small meals throughout the day, rather than relying on three, larger meals. Choose healthy options every few hours to keep hunger at bay and optimize your metabolism.

Get Support from Others

Remember that there are others that are in the same boat. Whether you join a support group, get involved in an online chat room, or create a circle of friends with a common goal, you can always find someone to help you avoid binge eating. Make sure you have someone you can call when you are about to give in. It's always helpful to have a steadfast friend or mentor who will talk you down when you're ready to go on an eating spree.

Keep Yourself Busy

The last thing you need is too much down time. Go places and do things in your spare time. Don't allow yourself the opportunity to sit and think about food. Go hiking, take a day trip, or try a new hobby. Don't let the grass grow beneath your feet and you won't even have time to indulge in binge eating anymore.

Sometimes one of the best strategies to overcome a habit or disorder is to take action. Try to implement at least one of these strategies in the next two weeks and see how it can begin to change your life. Then, incorporate another strategy, until you have gained momentum toward recovery and positive changes in your life.

Chapter 10. The A-C-C-E-P-T Method to Re-Design Your Life

The A-C-C-E-P-T Method is a thought-restructuring system designed to enable you think positively and decision-make appropriately. Once you begin the process of sweeping away the cobwebs of old thinking patterns, you may feel the urge to "redesign" your life. Think of it like this: it's time to update your thought patterns, much like you'd want to give an old house a new look. Using the acronym A-C-C-E-P-T as a blueprint, you can recreate your life:

A - Accept. Until we are able to admit we have a problem and can accept that we need support, we're stuck in denial. Instead of remaining powerless, ask the Power of your Higher Self for strength and direction. Some people call this spiritual and universal power "God." Others believe it is their conscience. Others do not relate to those concepts, but understand there is a part of them which believes they can overcome. I have a client who calls it his, "Wise Self." In my opinion, it doesn't matter what name you give it: just call on it in times of need, and be listening and open to its higher guidance and direction.

The surest way out of addictive behavior is to let someone in. While I think it's wonderful to ask a family member or friend into your circle, the #1 problem I see when treating addictions is that clients resist telling their story to people outside their comfort zone. This is a real predicament, because we don't always listen to the advice of family and friends-they are just "too close." And, we know (or hope) that they will keep loving us in spite of our weaknesses. It is trusting in our comfort-zones which have gotten us to the point of addiction in the first place, so staying in them is not going to help us climb out of them. This is where community comes in.

C - Create your life. The most powerful words that were ever uttered to me were these: "You are the creator of your life. You are the architect of your own life." The first part of my life was spent trying to please other people, and be who I was told I should be. You know what?

I didn't get very far, or produce very much, and I certainly wasn't very happy being who others told me I should be. To be genuinely happy, you must be yourself, 100% yourself. Once you have worked through the expectations of what other people want from you, and thrown that aside, you are in the unique position to begin living, really living.

To expect society, your cultural heritage, your parents, your company or your boss, your family or your partner to fulfill your life's purpose and destiny for you is to deny that you have that power. You may not feel like you're capable of starting life anew. You may not feel like you can rebuild and create something miraculous and amazing. But you also know that our feelings don't always tell us the truth. In fact, by reading this workbook, you have taken an important step in the right direction: you are becoming more self-aware every minute. There is a term in psychology called, "Internal Locus of Control." It describes people who understand that the power to create the outcome of their lives is internal, and not external. Then there are those who have an "External Locus of Control." These are the people who feel victimized and out of control. They feel life is circumstantial, it is environmental. Studies have shown that people with an Internal Locus of Control are by far happier and healthier than those who see themselves as victims of circumstance. The difference between these two outlooks is that people with internalized direction are people of action. They do not wait for someone to tell them which way to go. They are willing to take calculated risks, and to head towards their dreams, even if they are not sure exactly how it's going to unfold. They simply trust that when they get to the next fork in the road, they will know which way to turn. There is no other way to describe this state than to say these people have faith in themselves. They trust their ability to make decisions.

Here is a non-clinical definition of intelligence that really appeals to me: "Intelligence is the ability to respond well to change." Intelligent people do not fear change; instead, they leverage it to their advantage. They don't stick their heads in the sand and pretend. They see it coming and prepare for it. They say to themselves, "I never thought I'd be here, but here I am. How can I make the best of this situation?" That is an intelligent bird. When we give control to the automatic, addictive thoughts, we are accepting defeat; we are going down without a fight, which is why clients with addictions suffer with self-esteem issues. Clients express to me that there's a part of them which keeps telling them, hounding them that they can overcome the behavior, while a separate part of them believes that they are locked into an unbreakable pattern. In psychological terms, this is known as polarity of personality. All people do not suffer with addictive or compulsive behavior, but I assure you, we all share these two polarities of thought. Gestalt Therapy is founded on this understanding: all of us struggle inwardly with "doing the right thing." Hollywood has depicted this inward polarity as the devil sitting on one shoulder and an angel sitting on another shoulder, both whispering into your ear. To re-create your life, you have to be willing and determined to decide the course of your own destiny.

Life wasn't meant to be perfect. If you have perfectionist tendencies, let me remind you of something: Life is messy. In relationships, on the job, mistakes happen, because it is part of being human. Think of how a child learns: by its mistakes! You learned not to touch fire because you put your hand on something hot. Humans learn what to do by first learning what not do. In your quest for recovery should you have a slip and return to the addiction, go ahead and feel guilty for a few minutes, but then get over it. It's been my professional experience that it is the clients who stay mired and stuck in guilt and shame that relapse. That is, they completely stop trying and throw in the towel, due to a simple lapse. Please remember: a lapse is not a relapse. You're only defeated when you stop trying. I heard a minister wisely advise one time, "Never stop starting." When you have a lapse, remind yourself, "It's part of the recovery process. I have not failed if I start again. I'll just start over."

T - Thanks-Giving. All of us have something to be grateful for. Some of us have health, some have wealth, some have family, some have friends, some have fulfilling careers, some have comforting and loyal pets, some have faith in God...whatever you have, celebrate it. It was Oprah Winfrey who said, "You can have it all, you just can't have it all at once." Maybe someday you will have it all, and I hope you do. Until then, make it a daily ritual to practice being grateful for whatever small things you already have. Acknowledging the small things in our lives which are going well for us (even if it's as simple as a delicious cup of coffee) reminds us that life is not all bad. When we practice the power of gratitude, life seems to take on a more realistic and balanced perspective. If you make it a practice to celebrate the high points of your day, your attitude will improve, and people will enjoy your company more. Overall, a grateful person is a happy person.

Self-Intervention Exercises:

A-C-C-E-P-T

1. Accept Higher Insight

Write a statement of what you think your Higher Self or Wise-Self might say to you today about your recovery:

2. Creating Community

Write a statement that expresses what ideal community recovery support would look like for you, and why:

Write a statement expressing what you don't want in a community support program, and why:

Write a statement expressing what action steps you could take to find community support:

I could (list actions):

3. Create Your Life

A. What could you work on now that would make the biggest difference in your life? (Coping skills, medical intervention, communications within relationships, etc.):

B. For your life to be ideal, what are a few things that have to be different?

C. What would you try now if you knew you couldn't fail?

4. Everyone Stumbles

When you have a lapse, what is your action plan? (Removing Triggers, Urge Surf, Emergency Coping List, Chair Exercise/Reparenting, etc.)

A. Rate your level of willingness to find support in a lapse (0-10, 0=will not and 10=certain I will):

B. What are a few pro-active steps you could take to avoid being triggered?

5. Positive

A. What do you hope happens, or what are your expectations? What is the logical next step in your growth?

B. What post-traumatic growth can you identify that has taken place in your life as a result of your problem? (Example: "My problem has taught me to...")

C. What specific self-intervention exercises will you practice to further your post-traumatic growth? (Positive affirmations, body awareness exercises, mind-awareness exercises)

6. Thanks-Giving

A. What strengths do you possess?

B. What resources do you have in your environment which could assist you in attaining your recovery goals?

C. Who would you like to thank for the contribution they've made in your life? List them below, and how they have helped you:

Write any other thoughts about your process here:

Conclusion

When it comes to overcoming binge eating disorder, no case is identical or recovery going to be the same journey for everyone.

As you've read, maybe you've noticed certain behavior patterns within yourself, or others you know that may reflect binge eating disorder. The next step is to take action and seek treatment. Recovery is a journey and will not happen overnight, but with a small step of faith, you or your loved one can make a change to break free from compulsive eating.

We've looked at three of the most common underlying money misconceptions that are probably getting in the way of a money lifestyle that truly serves you. We've looked at some of the hidden beliefs that may be quietly limiting your ability to use money for what it is: a tool that can help you achieve your goals and create a life that fits with your values and principles.

Let's take a more practical look at your actual budget now, but try to keep in mind this bigger picture. Below we're going to look at ways to bring your actual spending habits closer in line with what's important to you. We'll look at ways to take the insanity out of spending and get a greater sense of control and awareness over how you use your money. You can follow the outline suggested below as often as you like. And since money advice is only good advice if it actually works for your life, feel free to adapt and adjust it as necessary.

Step One - Take a good hard look:

If you haven't already, it's time to look at what you spend in a typical month. You'd be surprised how few people know exactly what they spend and where. In fact, if you're hesitant to even look properly, ask yourself if there's something you're trying to avoid looking at too closely.

You can appraise your monthly spending in a few ways: looking at bank statements and going through each item carefully, highlighting every expense according to the type (eating, entertainment, clothing, schooling, debt etc.) is an easy and obvious way to start. You might like to download a money management app that will allow you to look at your expenses in a variety of ways – sometimes graphs and pie graphs really drive the point home.

Look at what percentage of your total income you're spending on each area (i.e. 30% on rent, 10% on food), look at savings and if you can, try to identify any long term trends (i.e. your rent keeps going up but your salary is staying the same, or you keep going into debt every January after Christmas).

It's just data at this point so try to stay curious and pretend it's someone else's spending you're looking at. If something feels too scary or depressing to look at, that's your cue to look even closer at it...

Step Two - Rate how well this budget is suiting your needs:

As we've seen, most money management advice out there has a very simplistic take on budgets: more money is good, less is bad. But I hope you've been convinced now to look at your budget with higher expectations.

Look at your spending habits in all their glory. Look at that awkward lump of debt you'd rather not think about. Look at your salary, what you (really!) spend on gym, on internet, on coffee and snacks, on medical expenses. Whether you did this exercise in full or merely thought about it, try to remember now what your ultimate values are as a human being, and what your achievements in life thus far have been.

Now, ask yourself, are your spending habits helping or hindering you in these values and achievements? Are you spending in alignment with these ideas – or in direct opposition to them?

Look for areas where you bleed a lot of money into things you don't actually care about. If you only buy a coffee and a snack every day at work because you're bored and unfulfilled, you're spending inefficiently. If you can identify where you are trying to "buy your emotions," then you can cut that spending and think of real ways to address that emotional need – you'll help yourself and save that cash all at the same time.

You may notice that wasting a hundred dollars each month on expensive coffee and treats during lunch hour is just a small thread – but pull on it and you may discover it leads to bigger lifestyle changes you might be ready for. You may discover that overspending in this area only happens because you're bored with your job and need to ask for more challenging projects. This may be just the impetus to admit that it's time to ask for a promotion or look for another job. Had you merely tried the standard budgeting advice (buy a coffee machine for home instead and take it work in a thermos! Have tea instead, it's cheaper!) you've gone a step further and made meaningful changes to your lifestyle.

Take a moment to look and see whether your spending habits and attitude to money is doing its job of helping you achieve your goals.

Step Three - Re-prioritize:

That's fine. Without changing your total income or your total expenditure, attempt now to reshuffle and put your resources to their best possible use. Is your lifelong goal of learning to play the violin more important than wasting hours every evening binge watching series? Then stop paying for TV each month and funnel that money instead into a fund for violin lessons. If you value the idea of making meaningful change in the world, or of doing the right thing, cut that useless gym membership you keep paying for and offer to volunteer at a dog shelter instead. You still get some exercise, you save money and you do something that's ultimately worth so much more to you.

Think creatively here. Don't assume you "need" something. Ask yourself honestly if you just want it. Some choices can be difficult of course, and most of us are working with very limited incomes. But make this easier for yourself by contextualizing: going to the movies every weekend feels indispensable …but is it more valuable to you than paying down that depressing debt?

When you use your deepest values as your yardstick, these choices become easier. It may feel miserable to trim down your food or eating budget, but it may energize you to make those same cuts if you know that the money you're saving is going towards buying a gift for someone you love, or for the holiday of a lifetime, or your child's education. The great thing about editing your budget according to your own values is that you're not making or saving more money, but using the money you already have to its best purpose. You're optimizing. And so you don't have to feel miserable forcing yourself to be frugal, because your actions are naturally geared towards a lifestyle that means something to you. You're not trimming your budget, you're enriching your life. You're not taking away, but adding.

Step Four - Develop active habits:
All the money epiphanies in the world mean nothing until they're put into action. The whole point of looking closely at your spending habits, your money psychology and the misconceptions fueling your spending habits is simple: do something about it.

Thankfully, the smallest changes are sometimes the best. Don't worry about making grand one-time gestures to fix up your money troubles once and for all. Rather, focus on small, realistic habits that you can do each and every day. It's these changes, after all, that will accumulate and go to making up the bulk of the life you want to create.

Let's say you commit to dropping expensive dinners with your partner. Many of us just default to eating as entertainment – but there's so much more to life than eating! Instead spend that money on things that you both actually enjoy: buy board games, save up for a hobby you can both do together or go to interesting talks or workshops. Instead of taking public transport, take your bike and you save money and get some fitness into your schedule at the same time.

Here's a more extreme example. Let's say you look at your budget and realize that although you deeply value travelling and learning about new and exciting places, you haven't actually been able to afford a real holiday for years. But you fritter away money every year on travelling to visit distant family members, people who you don't like much and who don't seem to like you either. Not only do these family members add nothing to your life, they actively make you less happy by adding stress and keeping you from putting that money towards a trip that would actually make you happy.

Just by looking realistically at your budget, you've discovered that you have also been spending too much time on unfulfilling relationships that are more about obligation than anything else. Without spending an extra cent, you make it a habit to treat yourself each year to a weekly vacation somewhere you want to go.

Step Five - Rinse and repeat:
As we've seen, happy spending habits are more or less always a work in progress. Make daily changes to your life and try on new habits for size. Then have another look and ask how those changes are working for you. Can you change something else? Is there something new you've learnt? Have you learnt how not to do it?

Tips on Surviving a Money Crazy World:
Avoid, wherever you can, the temptation to spend on impulse. If you always give yourself a "cooling off period," you'll minimize emotional spending or buying something just because of sneaky advertising. For smaller purchases, wait 24 hours, and for bigger purchases, sleep on it for a few days before committing.

When you're spending money on something, don't focus only on the price you see in front of you. Ask yourself what this item really costs you. How long did you have to work to afford it? By working that long and exchanging that time for money for this item, did you really get a "good deal"? Could you use that time or that money on something else, that's worth more to you? Is that money actually worth more unspent, i.e. do you really have to buy anything at all?

Fast forward purchases a few years. Many of us throw away huge amounts of junk from our homes every year, and also keep buying things obsessively, never making the connection between the two. Are you going to get bored of this item within a few months? Will it really last? How will it fit into your life? Are you actually just buying next year's junk?

Don't go to shopping malls unless you're feeling calm, rational and in control. This means avoiding the shops when you're hungry, sad, bored, angry... You'll only be extra susceptible to advertising and pressure to "buy solutions." You'll have to work extra hard to resist temptation and may fall into the trap of feeling that you're depriving yourself.

Be prepared. It's so much easier to act wisely when you're acting according to a plan you've spent time on beforehand. Know how much you can afford to spend on a night out before you leave. Go shopping with a list and don't buy anything not on that list. Pack a work lunch the night before so you're not tempted to buy something expensive on the spur of the moment when you get hungry.

Try to see if you can spend your money on lived experiences rather than things. Things get old. They break. People get bored of them. But happy memories can last a lifetime, and if your experience teaches you a new skill or gives you a fresh insight on life, even better. Think of travelling somewhere novel, seeing a show, going to a class to learn something new, challenging yourself to a marathon or climb, donating to a charity that means something to you, experiencing beautiful music or performances, going into nature ...all of these things have so much more value compared to something like a phone upgrade or a new piece of furniture for your home.

Carry only small amounts of cash on you, for emergencies. This will deter you from spending mindlessly. It's easy to think of a few coins in your wallet as nothing much, but they add up. Spending on bank cards has the added advantage of letting you track exactly how much and on what you spend your money.

If you're trying to develop your professional career, you might like to consider negotiating for and working towards a higher hourly rate with less total time worked rather than endlessly angling for more work. In the long term, you'll value your time more and more. As you upskill and become more experienced, look for more job flexibility, more benefits and more free time rather than just a higher salary. Employers are usually a bit happier to negotiate on these anyway, and they'll actually have a greater impact on your quality of life.

When making big spending decisions, consider how a choice will mature with time. It may be that it's better to spend on X rather than Y in the present moment, but wait ten years and X just gets worse and worse as a choice. When considering big purchases, spending on education or paying off debt, ask yourself what will give you the greatest flexibility and control in the future. Ask which choice gives you more choices later on. Give less weight to choices that can't be undone or modified and more weight to those that can.

Don't be afraid to talk about money. Let go of hang ups and ask for help and advice when you need it. There's no shame in having money difficulties or being stuck with debt – but it's a real shame if you let hang ups about money prevent you from tackling a serious problem head on.

Some of our most nonsensical spending habits are closely tied with our worst life habits in general. Do you have an unhealthy drinking or smoking habit? This is the kind of thing you pay for over and over again – you pay for the substance itself, you pay with diminished health and you may even have to pay later on for medicine or treatment for health problems you bring on yourself. When it comes to any kind of addiction, it's never worth it. If this is you, the best thing you can do for yourself is clean up this bad habit. Drop your nasty sugar addiction. Quit smoking. Cut back on drinking. Vow to stay away from junk food.

Avoid comparing yourself to others. There's a lot of ego bound up in money, and it's hard to break the automatic connection that money = success. If you're suffering from trying to keep up with your peers, try to remember that people willfully display the life they want you to see, and there are invariably problems that you never know about. Keep going towards your own goals. If someone's success feels intimidating, try turn that feeling into inspiration – how can you do the same? What can you learn from them?